TEACHING INPATIENT MEDICINE

Dear Joy,
   Lovely to meet you.
        Best regards,
         Nate Houk

Dear Joy —
Great to meet you and
Go BLUE !!

Teaching Inpatient Medicine

What Every Physician Needs to Know

MOLLY HARROD, PHD

SANJAY SAINT, MD, MPH

WITH

ROBERT W. STOCK

OXFORD
UNIVERSITY PRESS

Oxford University Press is a department of the University of Oxford. It furthers the University's objective of excellence in research, scholarship, and education by publishing worldwide. Oxford is a registered trade mark of Oxford University Press in the UK and certain other countries.

Published in the United States of America by Oxford University Press 198 Madison Avenue, New York, NY 10016, United States of America.

Library of Congress Cataloging-in-Publication Data
Names: Harrod, Molly, author. | Saint, Sanjay, author. | Stock, Robert W., author.
Title: Teaching Inpatient Medicine : What Every Physician Needs to Know / Molly Harrod, Sanjay Saint, Robert W. Stock.
Description: Oxford ; New York : Oxford University Press, [2017] | Includes bibliographical references and index.
Identifiers: LCCN 2016043763 (print) | LCCN 2016044863 (ebook) | ISBN 9780190671495 (pbk. : alk. paper) | ISBN 9780190671501 (UPDF) | ISBN 9780190671518 (e-pub)
Subjects: | MESH: Education, Medical | Internship and Residency—standards | Group Processes
Classification: LCC R737 (print) | LCC R737 (ebook) | NLM W 18 | DDC 610.71/1—dc23 LC record available at https://lccn.loc.gov/2016043763

This material is not intended to be, and should not be considered, a substitute for medical or other professional advice. Treatment for the conditions described in this material is highly dependent on the individual circumstances. And, while this material is designed to offer accurate information with respect to the subject matter covered and to be current as of the time it was written, research and knowledge about medical and health issues is constantly evolving and dose schedules for medications are being revised continually, with new side effects recognized and accounted for regularly. Readers must therefore always check the product information and clinical procedures with the most up-to-date published product information and data sheets provided by the manufacturers and the most recent codes of conduct and safety regulation. The publisher and the authors make no representations or warranties to readers, express or implied, as to the accuracy or completeness of this material. Without limiting the foregoing, the publisher and the authors make no representations or warranties as to the accuracy or efficacy of the drug dosages mentioned in the material. The authors and the publisher do not accept, and expressly disclaim, any responsibility for any liability, loss or risk that may be claimed or incurred as a consequence of the use and/or application of any of the contents of this material.

1 3 5 7 9 8 6 4 2

Printed by Webcom, Inc., Canada

To my greatest teachers, Troy, Ben, and Ava Demo
Molly Harrod

*To the 12 superb attending physicians highlighted in this
book who allowed us to learn so much from them*
Sanjay Saint

To Jack
Robert W. Stock

CONTENTS

PREFACE

Our book—*Teaching Inpatient Medicine: What Every Physician Needs to Know*—is aimed at those who want to become better inpatient attending physicians. Medical education on the wards must, increasingly, be high yield given recent resident work duty restrictions and the imperative to deliver high-quality and efficient care. This educational responsibility falls on the shoulders of the attending physicians, men and women who have been educated themselves in the system, few of whom have had any formal education in teaching.

Attendings must teach more than the scientific knowledge and the technical skills necessary to deliver quality care. Physicians in training must learn how to communicate with patients, family members, and other healthcare providers; they must learn professionalism, time management, and how to be independent while an active member of a team. To provide high quality and value to patients, we must ensure that physicians in training are provided high quality and value in their clinical education. The recent shift from a physician-centric model of care to a patient-centered model of care requires physicians to communicate and interact with individuals they may not have collaborated with in the past. Attending physicians, who may have been educated under the old model, now have to teach the next generation how to deliver care that is team-based and patient-centered.

The successful attending physician will also have constraints on her time. Not only is she responsible for the medical team but, first and foremost, for patient care. Attendings in the 21st century care for more complex patients, have more interactions with other healthcare providers in the hospital (e.g., consulting physicians, radiologists, pharmacists, social workers, discharge planners), and spend more time on documentation, not to mention the continued responsibilities of the work they do when not attending on the wards.

Yet with all of these competing and challenging aspects of clinical training, this system of clinical education remains the cornerstone of preparing the next generation of physicians. As might be expected, the quality of the teaching that attendings provide is varied: some are great, others less so. What makes one more successful than another? We believe that there are opportunities to learn from those who are considered outstanding teachers. By studying how highly regarded attendings manage the complexity of the wards, both junior attendings as well as those more established can learn a great deal.

Although a good amount of research has focused on how clinical teachers approach the learning environment and what they do within those boundaries, these studies tend to focus on only one perspective (students or teachers). They often do not take into account multiple perspectives on the same team or in the same study (e.g., focus is on medical students or interns) nor do they look at the role allied health professionals and patients have in the learning process. To understand teaching as a lifelong process, we must go beyond asking what personal attributes an attending should have and instead ask what type of learning environment the best attendings create and how they manage and change this environment as different emphases on patient care emerge. Thus, it has become necessary to return to the wards to once again understand how the next generation of physicians is learning to care for patients. Therefore, we embarked on a journey to better understand:

1. What types of environments do great medicine attendings create?
2. How do great medicine attendings create these environments?
3. How do they teach multilevel learners to provide exceptional inpatient care?

We sought to use our findings to help guide other attendings who are looking for ways to improve their teaching approach.

The book is the work of a medical anthropologist with expertise in using qualitative techniques in healthcare settings, an academic physician with a long-standing interest in medical education who serves as a ward attending and oversees a medical service, and a journalist/book author with a specialization in medical topics. The book is written to be conversational in style and rich in practice-based anecdotes. While the primary audience is the attending physician who wishes to improve, either a recent graduate from a training program or one with more experience on the wards, medical educators, inpatient directors, and physicians-in-training may also find our findings and recommendations useful.

There are many people who helped bring this book to fruition. First and foremost, we would like to thank the attendings and their teams (both current and former) who welcomed us into a "day in their life" and shared with us their time, knowledge, thoughts, and experiences. It goes without saying that this book would not have been possible without all of you. Second, a huge thank you to Karen E. Fowler who planned, organized, and kept the research on schedule. Third, thank you to Jason Mann who helped with the final preparations of the book. And, finally, to our families, who saw us off on each site visit fully supportive of the work we were doing.

We hope you enjoy reading the book as much as we have enjoyed preparing it.

Molly Harrod, PhD
Sanjay Saint, MD, MPH
Robert W. Stock

ABOUT THE AUTHORS

Molly Harrod, PhD, is a trained medical anthropologist with the VA Ann Arbor Center for Clinical Management Research. She has been involved in numerous qualitative and mixed-methods studies focusing on such topics as clinician communication and teamwork, behavior change, patient safety, and implementation science. In addition, she has trained other health researchers in qualitative methods including semi-structured interviewing and the use of observation in research.

Sanjay Saint, MD, MPH, is the Chief of Medicine at the VA Ann Arbor Healthcare System and the George Dock Professor of Internal Medicine at the University of Michigan. His research focuses on patient safety and clinical problem-solving. He is a special correspondent to the *New England Journal of Medicine* and an editorial board member of the *Annals of Internal Medicine.* He received his Medical Doctorate from the University of California at Los Angeles (UCLA), completed a medical residency and chief residency at the University of California at San Francisco (UCSF), and obtained a masters in public health (as a Robert Wood Johnson Clinical Scholar) from the University of Washington in Seattle. He received the 2016 Mark Wolcott Award for Clinical Excellence from the Department of Veterans Affairs as the National VA Physician of the Year, and he was recently inducted into the Royal College of Physicians in London as an Honorary International Fellow.

Robert W. Stock is a freelance book and magazine writer. As an editor, writer, and columnist for *The New York Times* for three decades, and as a freelancer, he has frequently written about medical subjects ranging from amniocentesis to genetic counseling to public health.

1

Teaching Medicine

■□■

Example is not the main thing in influencing others. It is the only thing.

—ALBERT SCHWEITZER

THE MEDICAL STUDENT wanted to refer one of his patients to his attending physician who had an outpatient clinic, but the attending shook his head. "Because of logistical and political reasons, I can't see him," he said. Then he continued: "I hope you were referring him to me because you thought I could help and not because we both have the same strong personality and you think it would be a good fit."

The attending could simply have said no, period, leaving the student feeling confused and/or embarrassed. Instead, he offered an explanation for his decision—and then used humor to diffuse the situation.

There was a time in the history of clinical education when an abrupt and uninformative "no" would have been a familiar reaction to the student's suggestion. In those days, attending physicians were the largely unquestioned lords of the hospital. The state of medicine was such that they personally could provide for most of their patients' hospital care, and they expected unlimited hours and total commitment from their learners. It could be a brutal apprenticeship, but it produced generations of dedicated, efficient practitioners.

Gradually, and then in a rush over the past few decades, the medical world in general and hospitals in particular have undergone seismic change. Today's attendings and learners are part of a very different and far more complex and demanding hospital environment. Medical education has never been so challenging.

This book is designed to help attending physicians meet that challenge. The attending referred to at the start of this chapter is one of 12 carefully selected, exemplary physician teachers from around the country whom the authors observed making rounds on their hospitals' wards. The 12 were also interviewed—as were their current team members (medical students, interns, and residents)—as were some of the practicing physicians who had once been team members of the 12. By means of this multifaceted, in-depth exploratory, qualitative approach, we have been able to describe just how these great attendings go about creating an inspiring, effective learning environment tailored to the vastly altered requirements of the 21st-century hospital.

What makes this book particularly valuable for attending physicians, we believe, is that it goes beyond the listing of desirable teaching attributes that most previous studies have offered. It provides a close-up, detailed description of the specific strategies, methods, and even language that the 12 outstanding physicians use in their interactions with learners and patients on the wards.

Medical schools that are members of the Association of American Medical Colleges (AAMC) now graduate some 16,000 students a year. Most of these students will continue their medical education at one of the more than 1,000 teaching hospitals.[1] AAMC-member institutions, although just 6% of all hospitals, provide 71% of all level-one trauma centers, 61%

of pediatric intensive care units, and 35% of all hospital charity care.[2] They are intense environments. There, along with some graduates of international medical schools, the learners will be handed over to a series of attending physicians who have had little or no training in the art of teaching and who must navigate a perfect storm of pressures and distractions.

Advances in medical knowledge and technology have made it nearly impossible for any single physician to handle a patient's care today. Attendings now function as part of a team that includes nurses, pharmacists, radiologists, and other specialists. Dr. Elias Zerhouni, a former director of the National Institutes of Health, has estimated that the number of clinical staffers working with a single hospital patient soared from about 2.5 in 1960 to 17 or more in 2006.[3]

Teamwork calls for personal qualities such as empathy and communication skills that were not especially emphasized among attendings in previous generations. Moreover, the old physician-centered model of hospital care has yielded to a patient-centered model. Hospitals now list patient satisfaction alongside high-quality healthcare as one of their primary goals. Attendings and learners explain diagnoses and treatments to patients and their families and incorporate patients' views into treatment decisions.

The time pressure on today's attending physicians is unprecedented. As in years past, they must care for their own patients in addition to their teaching responsibilities and any other work they have when not attending on the wards. But now, as the general population has aged, attendings are treating patients with far more complex problems—and this at a time when hospitals are discharging patients sooner than ever before. Attendings and their teams have less time to spend with individual patients who, by and large, need more time. Patients who might have stayed in the hospital for several weeks in earlier times, giving learners a chance to become familiar with their medical issues and treatment outcomes, now leave in a matter of days. The time spent in bedside rounding, an indispensable element of a clinical education, has shrunk, while the hours devoted to organizational matters, record keeping, and quality improvement projects have multiplied.

As a demonstration of how administrative activities can interrupt learning: When we were accompanying one of the 12 attendings on rounds, an intern had to step away several times to answer a page about a patient transfer. When team members get pulled away to deal with "administrative stuff," the attending said, "It drives me nuts!"

In an effort to prevent medical errors by exhausted learners, the resident work week was lowered to 80 hours in 2003, and a shift cap of 16 hours for interns was instituted in 2011. The moves have substantially increased the time pressure on both attendings and learners. The learners now have fewer hours in which to shoulder the same workload—and the attendings have less instruction time to impart an ever more complex body of medical knowledge. The compression of the learners' hours has also inspired frequent schedule adjustments. As a result, the members of an attending's team may vary from day to day, depriving them of the essential experience of caring for a single group of patients and breaking the continuity of the attending's instruction.

The changes of recent years have drastically complicated the task of being an attending physician, and that is especially difficult for those who were trained under the old physician-centric regimen. As teachers, they must now be exemplars of 21st-century hospital medicine for their learners, role models for the delivery of team-based and patient-centered care.

Over the years, the vital importance of clinical education has inspired dozens of studies aimed at measuring the effectiveness of various teaching programs and offering recommendations for how best to do the job. Most of the studies provide lists of personal attributes and approaches to teaching that are favored by current learners based on their answers to questionnaires. Often, these inquiries fail to take into account the individual learner's level of education— medical students, for example, tend to place a high value on attendings who are nice to them, whereas residents want attendings who will give them maximum autonomy.[4,5] In other inquiries, the work of attendings is observed and analyzed by other physicians. But both varieties of study rely on just a single perspective, and neither looks at teaching as a practice that utilizes other allied health professionals or patients in the learning process.

In the past decade, there have been relatively few publications—books or journal articles—that examine the new circumstances of attending physicians and their efforts to adapt. This book was created to help fill that vacuum. In it, we ask three pivotal questions: What kind of learning environments do great attendings create? How do they create these environments? And, how do they teach multilevel learners to provide exceptional inpatient care?

To find the answer, we began with the assumption that teaching of any kind is a social process in which the students are active participants, not simply passive recipients of knowledge. Through that ongoing interaction, attendings and their team members create a community of ideas, values, and meanings that eventually yields an in-depth understanding of their shared world.[6] To discover how this process functions at the highest level, we began by seeking out great attending physicians—specifically, those who rounded on a general medicine floor regardless of their medical specialty. If we could really capture their educational methods, we believed that we could provide a uniquely helpful guide for other attendings.

Since there is no national ranking of attending physicians, we asked for nominations from two basic sources: The chiefs of medicine or other high-level officials at some of the nation's leading medical schools, and individual experts who had won teaching awards or were medical education specialists. Medical schools, excellence aside, vary in their resources and in the backgrounds of their students, and we made sure our school selections reflected those facts.

Once we had 59 attending nominees, we narrowed the list, seeking to make sure that a diversity of backgrounds (e.g., gender, ethnicity) and attending experience would be represented in our final grouping. That left 16 possible participants, and 12 of them agreed to take part in our study— not a small commitment on their part.

They would have to put up with us as observers and note-takers as they made ward rounds with their teams. They would have to sit down for individual interviews with us. And they would help us arrange to have further interviews with their current learners and with some of their former learners. We, in turn, agreed that our observations and the participants' comments included in this book would not be identified with any individual person. Their participation, though, is no secret: A photograph and brief biography of each can be found in the Appendix.

We should note that the 12 attendings were uncomfortable with the notion of themselves as "great" and only agreed to be part of our study because of its potential contribution to the field. During our interviews with them, they all suggested other physicians we should be studying. Indeed, we were very conscious of the fact that our list of great attendings leaves out hundreds of outstanding attendings all across the country.

Social processes are hard to pin down, and the work of the attending physician is no exception. This study utilized an in-depth exploratory, qualitative approach.[7] To understand the behavior and culture of these clinical teams, we spent time with their members in the context of their daily lives, going on rounds with them. In addition, our interviews provided multiple perspectives on the 12 attendings' modus operandi. The interviews with the attendings revealed their own views of the most important methods they use. Interviews with current learners provided evidence of how the attendings' methods were perceived by their most important audience. The comments of physicians who had been taught by the 12 attendings gave us an insight into the long-term effects of the attendings' approach. In all our dealings within the hospital setting, by the way, we had a distinct advantage: We were familiar with the territory. One of our team members is a physician who frequently attends on the wards and serves as chief of medicine, and another is a medical anthropologist who has conducted multiple studies in these settings.

In this book, we have organized the attributes and methods of the 12 attendings into several categories, starting with a general description of them as a group. We then show how the attendings create a team environment and a supportive learning environment; how they teach; and how they work with patients. At the end of each chapter we itemize its main points and provide suggestions for further reading on these topics. A final chapter summarizes our key findings.

Fair warning: We have not included ambulatory care in our research. We believed that there was a particular need for in-depth research into on-the-wards medical instruction in the transformed hospital setting and that our particular skills and backgrounds were more oriented in that direction. In addition, the inpatient and ambulatory settings emphasize different aspects of patient care. Because of this, we think that teaching in the ambulatory realm deserves its own study.

During our research, we saw that some techniques and personal qualities of the 12 attendings were at work in more than one aspect of their calling. A sense of humor, for example, was invaluable with both learners and patients. But the ways in which the attendings exercised their sense of humor differed considerably—self-deprecating, for example, versus joking. In the pages that follow, we illustrate with examples from our observations and recordings just how the attendings use their sense of humor as well as their other attributes and skills. It is in those very details, we believe, that readers will find the special contribution of this book.

It should be noted that, in some cases, the transcripts of interviews with attendings and learners have been edited for length and clarity. Also, not all of the behaviors and techniques presented in the book were exhibited by every one of the 12 attendings. Instead, we have chosen to highlight various aspects of teaching and patient care that many of the learners and attendings emphasized as being effective and necessary in today's healthcare environment.

Finally, each chapter is organized similarly. It will begin with a quote that exemplifies a key idea that will be discussed. Each chapter will also end with three main points that the reader should take away from the chapter. Finally, for those interested in learning more, we suggest several references for further reading, along with annotations.

MAIN POINTS

1. Time constraints, complex patients, and the involvement of multiple disciplines in the care of patients have necessitated changes in medical education on the units.

2. Unlike prior research, this project focused on the context in which learning happens and selected the team as the focus of research.

3. We spent time with 12 attendings and their teams in order to provide detailed descriptions of the specific strategies, methods, and even language that the attendings use to teach their learners not only about medicine in general but also about how to care for patients.

Further Reading

Wachter, R. M., & Verghese, A. (2012). The attending physician on the wards: Finding a new homeostasis. *Journal of the American Medical Association, 308*(10), 977–978.

   In this viewpoint, the authors, national leaders in academic medicine, present a picture of how the role and responsibilities of the attending have changed over time. They compare the teaching approach of older versus younger attendings and make the point that systems changes are necessary to accommodate these new approaches and requirements. For example, they emphasize that institutions should provide the support necessary to ensure a balance between teaching and providing patient care.

Asch, D. A., & Weinstein, D. F. (2014). Innovation in medical education. *New England Journal of Medicine, 371*(9), 794–795.

An Institute of Medicine report (Committee on the Governance and Financing of Graduate Medical Education: Graduate medical education that meets the nation's health needs) concluded that there is a fundamental lack of research in the area of medical education. The authors of this perspective call for research that would focus on developing and defining measures of training success, that would highlight the changes needed in the structure and content of medical education, and that would provide new models for financing medical education.

Stern, D. T., & Papadakis, M. (2006). The developing physician—Becoming a professional. *New England Journal of Medicine, 355*(17), 1794–1799.

In this review article, Stern and Papadakis state that educational and training environments have changed substantially in recent years and that it is time to re-evaluate the professional behaviors necessary to practice medicine in today's environment. The concept of teaching must include not only medical knowledge, but also three other basic categories: setting expectations of professionalism and defining what that means, providing experiences that will support the development of humanistic attitudes, and evaluating outcomes that include methods for measuring professional behavior.

2

Why Study Attending Physicians?

■□■

Choose a job you love, and you will never have to work a day in your life.

— CONFUCIUS

ON ONE LEVEL, the nine men and three women we observed and interviewed are a mixed bag. Some entered their training knowing they wanted to specialize in internal medicine, while others fell in love with the specialty during their training. One of the attendings started out in psychiatry and another in orthopedic surgery. Eight of them are former chief medical residents and seven did their residency in a hospital where they now work. One was inducted into his state's football hall of fame, while another was a medical school valedictorian.

The 12 also have their individual styles of doctoring and teaching that generally match up with their personalities. One is a walking sunbeam, greeting passersby in the hallways, constantly joking with his team. Another conveys her warmth and humor in a quieter but no less effective manner. During ward rounds, some attendings are more hands-on with patients than others; some spend more time and energy on table rounds than their counterparts.

Yet, for all such differences, the 12 share some basic qualities and attributes. Most of them, for example, are hospitalists, members of history's fastest growing medical specialty. Hospitals in Great Britain and elsewhere had employed inpatient physicians for years, but they were rare in the United States (U.S.) in 1996. That's when an article in the *New England Journal of Medicine*, authored by Drs. Robert Wachter and Lee Goldman from the University of California at San Francisco, coined the term "hospitalist" and called for a new and more efficient division of labor—hospitalists for inpatients, primary care physicians for outpatients.[1] That arrangement, the authors argued, would assure that there would always be doctors on hand to care for hospital patients in need while freeing up primary care doctors to spend more time with their outpatients.

The seed was planted. From that standing start two decades ago, the ranks of hospitalists have burgeoned to more than 40,000. They can be found in 70% of U.S. hospitals and not just as internists. Today, there are orthopedic hospitalists, neurological hospitalists, and obstetrics-gynecological hospitalists, to name a few. The hospitalist movement has been a key element in the transformation of American hospitals, aiding in the effort to shorten patients' stay and reduce costs. At the same time, hospitalists have played a crucial supporting role in the hospital industry's drive, under pressure from Washington and the public, toward higher quality, patient-centered care.[2]

The 12 attendings we studied are also very much alike in their full-hearted enthusiasm for their work. They are constantly striving to improve both their knowledge base and their teaching skills. And they have no hesitation admitting when they are wrong or simply don't know the answer to a learner's question.

This description of an attending by one of his former learners sums up the whole group: "No matter how many awards he might have won or how many other leadership positions he might have, ultimately, he was a doctor that loved taking care of patients and loved teaching—never there to sort of just get through something so that he could get on to something else, but very present and very excited about what he was doing."

Another of the 12 said of his calling, "I take great joy." He described the surprised reaction of hospital staffers when he showed up for work on a day off. "What are you doing here? It's Christmas." The attending's response: "I'm blessed. That's why I'm here."

Nothing is so powerful in accomplishing a challenging mission as a joyous commitment. As Steve Jobs put it, "The only way to do great work is to love what you do."

The 12 attendings' enjoyment of teaching grows, in part, from their interest in other people—particularly young people who are treading the same path the attendings chose for themselves. They take pleasure in getting to know their team members not just as the latest group of learners but as individuals, and conversations often extend beyond the world of the hospital.

All of the 12 attendings are highly intelligent, skilled, and knowledgeable physicians. "He just kind of knows a ton of [physical exam] maneuvers," a former learner said of his one-time attending, "some I have never even heard of. He just knows all of the data behind . . . the likelihood ratios for different things."

During the time they spend with their learners, the 12 are constantly looking for ways to share their knowledge (Figure 2.1). We observed attendings who simply never stopped teaching their teams—before rounds began, with the patients, walking from patient to patient (including a mini-lecture in a stairwell), and after rounds. They possessed information that could repair bodies and save lives, and they were determined to pass along as much of it as possible.

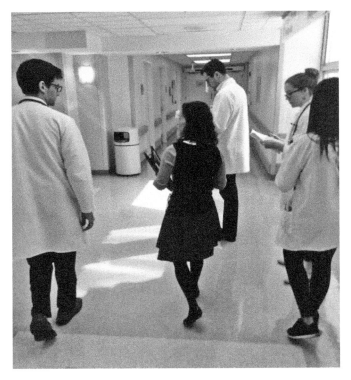

FIGURE 2.1 Attending physician utilizing every moment to teach.

Like anyone who loves his or her job, the 12 attendings are constantly alert for opportunities to do it better. They stay abreast of the medical literature and ferret out new facts wherever they are to be found. A former learner described his attending as "very curious," adding that he was "very much there to learn, to discover new things along with you." We heard one of the attendings telling his team that he had "checked the living daylights out of the literature" to follow up on a patient seen earlier. He finally decided to use a resource available to everyone: "I emailed the person that did the study and asked him about this." The upshot: "He said he's never seen this before."

Another attending asked one of his learners what he wanted to talk about. "I'm going into rheumatology," the learner told us, "so I did a little thing on vasculitis. And he sits there and takes notes." The teacher had no hesitation about becoming the learner. The next time anyone wants to know about vasculitis, the attending will have the answers.

As part of their determination to improve, the 12 attendings frequently gauge their own progress as well as that of their learners. One of them said he was "always thinking about what could have been done differently" after rounds were over. In this case, he was disappointed with himself for not being specific enough when he assigned some research. Self-assessment is a proven path. A 2015 study found that the more often you monitor your progress toward a goal, the more likely you are to succeed in attaining it.[3]

There are other attributes the 12 physicians have in common that will become apparent over the next chapters, but we would be remiss not to mention here their lightheartedness and their sense of humor. Often, their humor finds expression in quick asides. One of the attendings asked an intern if he could be more specific about the pathophysiology of a patient's problem. When the intern passed, the attending opened the question to the other members of the team: "Who's feeling more specific?" Self-deprecating humor is also popular. An attending urged her team to, "Talk to me like I know nothing." After a pause, she continued, "Thank you for not saying that's how you always talk to me."

And, occasionally, the attendings will channel their inner Jerry Seinfeld. We listened in as an intern, presenting a new patient, mentioned that the patient was receiving mineral oil enemas.

> ATTENDING: At home? If that's his significant other giving it to him, that's a pretty deep bond.
>
> INTERN: He's worried about morphine addiction. He has a history of it.
>
> ATTENDING: He should be worried about mineral oil addiction.

In the chapters ahead, we describe the team environment, the approach to teaching favored by the 12 attending physicians, and show the various methods they use to create and maintain that environment for each successive group of learners.

MAIN POINTS

1. Most of the attendings in this study are also hospitalists, specializing in the care of patients within the hospital.

2. Although each attending had his or her own individual style of doctoring and teaching, we were able to identify qualities and attributes they all shared.

3. One of the most important attributes all of the attendings shared was the conviction that they should never stop learning.

Further Reading

Wachter, R. M., & Goldman, L. (1996). The emerging role of "hospitalists" in the American health care system. *New England Journal of Medicine, 335*(7), 514–517.

> In this sounding board, the emerging role and potential future of the hospitalist in the American healthcare system is discussed. The authors describe the varying reasons why they believe the hospitalist specialist will flourish. They include cost pressures, the need for physicians who can provide care for a large panel of patients, and the ability of hospitalists to utilize immediately available resources to quickly respond to changes in a patient's condition. Wachter and Goldman also outline several objections facing the hospitalist model.

Rachoin, J. S., Skaf, J., Cerceo, E., Fitzpatrick, E., Milcarek, B., Kupersmith, E., & Scheurer, D. B. (2012). The impact of hospitalists on length of stay and costs: Systematic review and meta-analysis. *American Journal of Managed Care, 18*(1), e23–e30.

> In this systematic review and meta-analysis, Rachoin and colleagues pooled 17 studies to estimate the magnitude of the impact of hospitalists on length of stay and cost. They concluded that hospitalists significantly reduce patients' length of stay without increasing costs. They posit that their findings can be used to define and measure expectations of performance for hospital medicine groups.

Bennett, H. J. (2003). Humor in medicine. *Southern Medical Journal, 96*(12), 1257–1261.

> Despite statements that humor can result in health benefits, the author found that, given the current state of research, it is insufficient to validate such claims. Although tangible health

benefits were lacking, there was support in the literature for the roles that humor and laughter play in the areas of patient–physician communication, psychological aspects of patient care, medical education, and as a means of stress reduction in medical professionals.

3

Building the Team

■□■

You may have the greatest bunch of individual stars in the world, but if they don't play together, the club won't be worth a dime.

—BABE RUTH

THE ATTENDING PHYSICIAN, one of the outstanding 12, acknowledged that medical students can be extremely nervous when presenting in front of a patient for the first time. "But I think it is good for the patient," he said, "to know that all of our intellectual capital is focused on them, in that moment." He went on to compare what happened in the team presentations to the sharing of electrons in a chemical compound: "It's all about covalency. Most people are just working next to each other, not with each other."

All of the attendings told us, and showed us, how seriously they take their responsibility to establish and maintain that kind of team—cooperative rather than competitive, the members concerned for their patients and for each other. Such teams do a better job on the wards and a better job of learning to become outstanding doctors themselves. That double obligation to minister and to learn has a checkered history—as does the role of the attending physician.

Sadly, as Ken Bain[1] notes in his book, *What the Best College Teachers Do*, "teaching is one of those human endeavors that seldom benefits from its past. Great teachers emerge, they touch the lives of their students, and. . .

subsequent generations must discover anew the wisdom of their practices" (p. 3). But discover they do, and Bain concludes on a similarly positive note, convinced that "good teaching can be learned" (p. 21).

Back when the U.S. was born, doctors started as apprentices, gradually learning their masters' techniques for pulling teeth and bleeding the sick. Toward the end of the 18th century, the University of Pennsylvania medical school began providing a year of hospital study and clinical practice after completion of apprenticeship; it was the nation's first internship. Some would-be doctors were also able to further their study in Europe, which was far ahead of the U.S. in medical education.

The stage was set for the widespread development of university-sponsored, high-quality medical schools, with access to hospitals for clinical training on the charity wards. But, over the next century, as apprenticeship waned, a host of for-profit, ersatz medical schools popped up, most providing a bare modicum of classwork and little or no clinical experience. Graduates gained that experience on the backs, as it were, of their initial, unlucky patients. In a hint of better days to come, the Johns Hopkins Hospital opened in 1889 and was soon offering the nation's first residency for pursuit of specialty training, an opportunity that was reserved, however, for only the very top students. Medical school alone was no longer viewed as a sufficient preparation for practice.

As the country grew in the first years of the 20th century, the rapidly expanding hospitals relied more and more on house officers. They came cheap: Their primary reimbursement was room and board, which was how they came to be called residents. Over endless hours of the day, they performed many of the hospital's menial chores, but they were also learning. Time was set aside for interns and residents to examine patients and, especially at teaching hospitals, to treat them—all under the strict direction of the attending physician.

In 1914, the American Medical Association issued a list of 603 hospitals approved for the teaching of interns, and, over the next few decades, graduate medical education flourished. "Most faculty took a keen interest in teaching, advising, and mentoring," Kenneth M. Ludmerer says in his book, *Time to Heal*. "House officers could not help feeling close to—and supported by—their instructors."[2] It was, in fact, a reasonably sane environment with weeks for house officers to get to know and treat patients and without such modern pressure points as intensive care units.

After World War II, hospitals began a long period of exponential growth, spurred by government support and insurers' open-ended, fee-for-service payments. But, in the 1980s, Medicare and other insurers called a halt. Henceforth, hospitals would receive a fixed payment per patient depending on his or her diagnosis. The longer a patient remained in the hospital, the less likely it would be to recoup its expenses. So hospitals began shortening patients' stays—to the detriment of the house staff's training. Learners had less time with any given patient and, when their daily hours were limited in 2003, less time with their patients as a whole.

Teaching hospitals became more corporate, more intent on market share and cost efficiency. The close, supportive connection between attendings and learners was eroded as faculty applied for remunerative research grants at the expense of their teaching. Critics charged that house staff was spending fewer hours on the ward and at the bedside in favor of conference rooms and technological teaching aids. As a Boston University professor put it: "The wealth of bedside teaching opportunities is diminishing with rapid patient discharges, overabundance, and over-reliance on technology."[3]

The 12 outstanding attendings we followed know how to cope with the challenges of today's hospital. Their ability to build and maintain competent, cooperative teams is an essential part of that know-how.

At the core of their team-building skills is a firm determination to make it all about the team and to keep their own role to that of a watchful, benevolent coach. They have totally turned their backs on the physician-centric teams of the past. They see themselves as coaches more than bosses, since they expect the team to carry the ball with patients. Here's how one of them gets that message across:

> So when I sit down with the team, I ask them, "Who is in charge of this team?" And they all say, "You are." And I'll go, "No, it's [senior medical resident]. She's in charge of the team, and unless she decides to give someone heparin who has had an intracranial bleed, you have to do what she says, right? Otherwise, tape her to the chair and call me."

Our 12 attendings' approach to teaching is the very opposite of malicious pimping, the posing of purposefully esoteric, unanswerable questions by an attending to demonstrate his or her superiority. They want to encourage harmony within the group, not sow discord. In fact, when our 12 attendings ask questions of their teams, they are frequently pitched toward the lowest common denominator. "He would ask us questions that it would be clear the [medical] students would be able to answer," a former learner recalled. "It bred this environment of inclusion." For these attendings, every member of a clinical team is equal in terms of opportunities to learn, to carry the ball, and to teach.

One of the current learners described his attending's approach:

> The most junior person has to be in charge. The medical student is the one who is going into the room and asking the questions and doing the history and the physical. And when the attending comes in the afternoon and he wants to run the list, that medical student is the person who does it. It's not, you know, a five-minute job with the senior. It's everybody . . . taking care of their patients; they are in charge.

Being in charge, running bedside rounds in front of the attending, the patient, and the other team members, is a foundational learning experience, but the learning is not limited to the learner in charge. Team members benefit from discussions of the other members' patients, both the right calls and the mistakes. Attendings and patients benefit as well. "You are going to pick up on things for your patient that I won't pick up on," one attending tells his team.

Our 12 attendings want as many members of their team as possible to participate each day during rounds. For one thing, it allows attendings to evaluate how the various members are progressing in their clinical work. And having the team together on rounds builds cohesion. Members get to know each other better, share complaints and jokes, recognize strengths and weaknesses and allow for both (Figure 3.1). They help each other study, they have each other's back if there's a problem, they have fun. As legendary Michigan football coach Bo Shembechler would emphasize: "The team, the team the team."[4] A cohesive team, the attendings believe, does a better job of caring for patients.

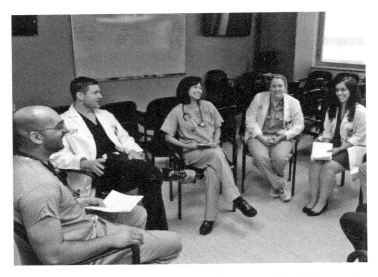

FIGURE 3.1 Members of a team getting to know each other before rounds.

One of the 12 described the outcome: "There is this incredible efficiency when the whole team sees the patient together and figures out the plan, and there is no 'I will see him later in the day' or 'We'll close the loop later on and see what the attending thinks.' We are done by 10:30 with our decision-making."

The team structure as a model for organizing work has in recent years won broad acceptance in industry. Studies have demonstrated that teams performing high-intensity tasks make fewer mistakes than individual workers. That comports with modern educational theory, which tends to identify two basic varieties of learning. The first is knowledge acquisition, enabling the individual to reproduce the information studied. The second variety is knowledge gained through participation in a dynamic community, a team; the individual's identity is altered in the learning process. Team learning has an obvious side benefit for hospitals where collaboration among clinicians (during resuscitation, for example) is so vital. And, as we noted earlier, clinical teams can bring more brainpower to bear on a patient's care than provided by a single practitioner. But the singular achievement of clinical team education, properly pursued, is the creation of principled, humane physicians who have absorbed the necessary knowledge and skills to practice good medicine.[5]

Each in his or her own way, the attendings start their team-building on the team's first day. One attending has the members write down three goals: (1) something they particularly want to learn about, (2) something they want to see fixed about the hospital, and (3) something personal they want to achieve. A former learner offered an example: "I will cook dinner five times during this rotation." The sharing of goals began the process of introducing the members to each other. It also, of greatest concern, alerted the attending to the members' clinical interests. Not least, the goals-gathering provided the attending with a team talking point for the future, as in: "Hey, Bill, how many of those dinners have you cooked so far?"

Another attending, at the first session with her team, stated some of her priorities, including her preference for short presentations at the bedside in the interest of efficiency. Then she asked the senior residents how they wanted to run rounds. What were some of the arrangements they liked or wanted to avoid? That led to a team discussion and a temporary consensus. "We've modified the plan over the last week and a half or so," a senior resident said, "to our own little version of what works best."

Some attendings make it a point to memorize the names of the team members the night before that first meeting. At the session itself, they make sure they are pronouncing the names correctly. One current intern reported, with amazement, that his attending actually got his name right—something few other attendings had bothered to master. Starting with the first meeting, the attendings make liberal use of the first person plural in referring to team activities. They say, "Why do we care?" It's "we," not "you," need to get the job done. Such small, tactful strategies go a long way toward creating a relaxed and collegial atmosphere.

Their personal styles and tastes dictate how the 12 attendings seek to put their teams at ease. One of them starts table rounds with music. On the day we visited, the attending selected Tom Petty's "The Waiting" because one of the team's interns was awaiting the birth of his first child. There was banter back and forth about The Eagles band, and it was very clear that team members were comfortable with the attending and with each other. It was also obvious that the attending knew what was going on in the members' personal lives as well as in their clinical lives.

As the coach, the attending has to guide and correct the learners in ways that will maintain their ability to do their work and protect team cohesion. We will describe some of those specifics in the next few chapters. But the single most important factor, the cement that holds a team together, is the members' trust in each other and in their attending physician. The development of that mutual trust is one of the 12 attendings' major goals. A current learner, for example, told us that his attending had primed the pump from the start: "You feel that he comes into the team trusting that you know what you are doing and that you care about your patients. You don't want to lose that."

Our attendings foster trust by demonstrating, day after day, that they will make sure the team's patients suffer no harm at the hands of the learners while, at the same time, the attendings give team members the greatest possible freedom to diagnose and treat those patients. They also build trust by creating a supportive environment, a place where team members feel they are safe to make a mistake or call for help. How they go about it is the subject of the next chapter. First, though, a look at how the 12 attendings work with nurses, pharmacists, radiologists, and other hospital personnel.

The resident and the pharmacist were talking in the hall outside a patient's room; the attending physician was still inside the room. At a crucial moment, the pharmacist had come up with some information about the patient the resident needed.

RESIDENT: Thanks for bailing me out.

PHARMACIST: No problem. Anytime.

ATTENDING: I heard that!

(Laughter all around.)

For most teaching settings, this would not be a typical encounter. According to a report summarizing the findings of a conference on the state of clinical education in the U.S., "In most teaching settings physicians learn and practice alongside nurses and other professionals, rather than with them."[6] That was not what we saw in our observations of the 12 attendings who treated other hospital personnel as ex officio members of their teams—"instead of having them just do our work," as one current learner put it. When a patient's nurse was nearby and not otherwise occupied, they asked the nurse to join in rounds. When pharmacists were part of rounds, their advice was sought and they were included in the team camaraderie. In addition, the attendings often led the team on forays to the radiology department, for example, asking personnel there to go over the radiographic findings from a recent study and do some teaching of their own.

In these encounters, our attendings were invariably attentive and respectful. As one of them told us, "I don't want the team to think that anything I have to say is more valuable than what our pharmacist or the nurses have to say." The attendings wanted the information these personnel could give the team, but they were also acting in their capacity as role models. Physicians, they were indicating, should treat all caregivers as colleagues, both because it's the proper thing to do and because it can help the physician do his or her job more efficiently. A failure of communication, so often the result of poor or non-existent relationships, is a major cause of preventable, hospital-based error.[7] And, from the attending's personal point of view, patronizing or otherwise "dissing" colleagues is an effective formula for failure.

"My default position about nurses," an attending told us, "is to respect their opinion as they have earned it. There are other nurses, I've learned their opinion doesn't mean as much, but I will still be nice to them. It's part of the collegiality, and I think it's important."

Some of the attendings routinely send a team member to find the nurse caring for the patient whom the team is about to visit. We listened as an attending asked a patient's nurse if she had any particular concerns to share with the team, then briefed her on the team's plan for the patient.

ATTENDING: Do you need anything from us?

NURSE: The patient said he wanted breakfast, so I called ultrasound and they said he could eat, but I wanted to check with you.

ATTENDING: Sure, if that's what they said.

ATTENDING: [TO PATIENT.] Good thing your nurse checked on that for you. Now we can get you some breakfast.

Throughout the entire encounter, the attending showed the nurse respect as a fellow professional caregiver and as a person. Praising her behavior to the patient served to strengthen the nurse's relationship with the patient *and* with the attending physician herself. By building positive connections with hospital personnel, the attendings find a particularly warm welcome when they take their teams to consult with those personnel.

That was definitely the case when we tagged along on a team visit to the radiology department. A resident radiologist pulled up the patient's images, and the team studied the film as the attending raised questions about it. The patient's images were then discussed by the attending radiologist, who was happy to show the team members some of the key elements in the film that pointed to a particular diagnosis.

To get the most out of what a former learner calls "interdisciplinary pit stops," one of the attendings has her team figure out what information the particular specialist will need. The former learner offered some examples:

If we want to consult nephrology for [acute kidney injury], what are they going to ask for? Are they going to ask for an ultrasound, are they going to ask for a urine study? Or if we were consulting neurology and we knew they were going to want a head MRI, we want to get that MRI done before we consult them. That way, it's more useful for them, and they can be ready for the next step.

In the next chapter, we show how our 12 attending physicians go about creating a supportive environment, one in which team members feel secure enough to accept and even welcome critical feedback as a necessary part of their path toward practice.

MAIN POINTS

1. The attendings used multiple strategies to build and maintain team relationships, such as acting as coaches allowing the learners to take the lead, trusting team members in the care of their patients, and getting to know the team members personally.

2. The attendings' definition of the team extended beyond the learners and included other allied health professionals.

3. Attendings view the care of a patient as the team's responsibility and not just that of the primary provider.

Further Reading

Cooke, M., Irby, D. M., Sullivan, W., & Ludmerer, K. M. (2006). American medical education 100 years after the Flexner Report. *New England Journal of Medicine, 355*(13), 1339–1344.

In this article, the authors summarize the changes in medical education over the past century and describe current challenges. The amount of medical knowledge has expanded at a time when the delivery of care has also become more complicated. The authors call for the use of various knowledge assessments to ensure that professional values, medical knowledge, and skills are attained.

Ludmerer, K. M. (1999). Instilling professionalism in medical education. *Journal of the American Medical Association, 282*(9), 881–882.

In this editorial, Dr. Ludmerer, an internationally renowned medical historian, provides an overview of the characteristics and factors that determine professionalism in the medical field. The author then goes on to explain the many pressures physicians face that impede their ability to put the patients' self-interest ahead of their own (a primary tenet of professionalism). To improve professionalism among physicians, Ludmerer suggests a broad-based approach focusing on formal coursework and faculty mentoring in addition to shifting the culture of academic and health centers from a focus on financial returns to one more service-oriented.

O'Leary, K. J., Buck, R., Fligiel, H. M., Haviley, C., Slade, M. E., Landler, M. P., . . . Williams, M. V. (2011). Structured interdisciplinary rounds in a medical teaching unit: Improving patient safety. *Archives of Internal Medicine, 171*(7), 678–684.

This article describes a study of an intervention designed to improve interdisciplinary collaboration and lower the rate of adverse events. The intervention, which took place in one of two medical teaching units in a tertiary-care academic hospital, combined a structured format for communication with a forum for regular interdisciplinary meetings. The authors found that structured interdisciplinary rounds significantly reduced the adjusted rate of adverse events.

4

A Safe, Supportive
Environment

■□■

*The greatest sign of success for a teacher is to be
able to say, "The children are now working as if I
did not exist."*

IN THE PREVIOUS chapter, we described team learning
as "knowledge gained through participation in a dynamic
community." But for a community to actually be dynamic,
there must be true collaboration.

Our 12 outstanding physicians achieve that team-oriented
goal in part by creating a climate in which learners feel it's safe
to flub a question or argue a diagnosis with their attending.
Learners discover that they and their ideas are valued and
that their mistakes are treated as learning opportunities—for
themselves and other team members. Moreover, our attendings also build relationships with individual team members,
providing support when learners encounter problems or
uncertainties, be they professional or personal.

This version of clinical education is a far cry from that
experienced by learners of earlier generations and by many
learners today. Too often, attending physicians on ward
rounds do more lecturing than listening. In our interviews of current and former learners, some spoke of being

criticized or demeaned by attending physicians in front of other people. As a current learner suggested, the impact can be lasting: "I think the first time you get shot down by an attending on rounds, especially like the first day or something, you're not going to say much more to that person for a while. Probably not going to have the courage."

That result is precisely what the 12 attendings want to prevent. Embarrassment, anxiety, and fear are enemies of rational thinking and the learning process. A substantial body of research supports the view that the most effective clinical education is collaborative rather than command and control, learning by doing rather than by rote and through lectures.[1] For their model to work, though, the attendings must gain the learners' trust, in part by trusting them to do their jobs. Attendings must also quickly acquire a sense of the needs and goals of the individual team members and strive to meet them. In other words, aside from an extensive knowledge base and clinical acumen, attendings need substantial people skills. As a review of the literature concerning the attributes of a good clinical teacher suggests, success "depends less on the acquisition of cognitive skills such as medical knowledge and formulating learning objectives, and more on inherent, relationship-based, non-cognitive attributes."[2]

Such attributes may be inherent for many people, but they are known as people *skills,* and, like other skills, they can be learned. In this chapter, we consider the approaches that the 12 outstanding attending physicians use to make team members feel safe and supported.

The behavior of the attendings toward team members and other hospital personnel established an environment that was welcoming and accepting. As both current and former learners told us with remarkable consistency, the attendings are generous with their praise for team members, especially the medical students and interns—those who generally need the most emotional reinforcement. It helps to create a positive atmosphere within the team. Sometimes the attendings' approval was expressed with a simple fist bump or a high five, sometimes with the simplest of words: "Good job," "Nice work," "Way to go," "That's exactly what I would do."

We witnessed the following exchange between one of our attendings and a resident:

ATTENDING: I thought you were going to get there. I was trying to lead you there.

RESIDENT: I know. [They high-five.]

ATTENDING: I like how proud you make me. It makes my heart warm.

The attendings' speech patterns and body language reinforced a supportive environment. Most of them spoke calmly and quietly. They were part of the circle during rounds, their eyes on the presenter, listening carefully and respectfully— they didn't answer pages (Figure 4.1). They seldom if ever interrupted a presentation, holding off any comments until it was finished; if seriously critical comments were necessary, they were generally delayed until they could be made to the presenter in private. On those occasions when the attendings did interrupt, it was to seek clarification, and it was done apologetically. As one of the attendings described his participation on rounds: "It takes us three or four days at the beginning of the month for people to understand to stop looking at me."

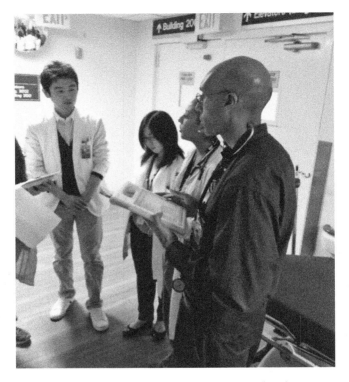

FIGURE 4.1 Senior resident leading rounds with attending listening in.

In their interactions with learners outside of rounds, the attendings presented themselves as open and accessible, easy to relate to, easy to talk to. They smiled. They maintained eye contact. There was no sense of impatience, no suggestion that they had to move on to more important matters. They were fully present. "When he's there, he's there," a learner said, "so there's nothing else on his mind." They treated the learners as colleagues.

The attendings also cultivated trusting relationships with their learners, engaging them in conversations about their interests outside the hospital. One of the attendings described his approach: "I say, 'Where are you from? Where did you go to high school? What did you do after college?' Invariably, the stories are great. You know, people have done amazing things."

At the same time, the attendings made it clear that they were ready and eager to help their team members when problems arose, day or night. On one level, of course, that is the basic, all-important requirement every attending demands of his or her learners: Contact me if you have any serious clinical doubts or problems you cannot handle. The knowledge that the attending is there for them at least partially relieves learners of their greatest fear, a mistake that could worsen a patient's condition or cost a patient her life.

Our 12 attendings also made sure their teams knew how to reach them 24/7. A former learner put it this way: "You can call him at 8 P.M. and he won't be pissed. He's like, 'Call me any time you have a problem; I'm ready to come on in and work it out with you guys.'" Many of the physicians rearranged their schedules for the time when they would be attending. "I try to decrease to only absolutely urgent meetings for these two weeks," an attending told us, "so I'm not distracted and can be available for them if needed." It's a crucial element of a safe and supportive environment.

On another level, the 12 attendings also made themselves available to help with nonclinical problems or concerns that were unique to individual team members. Sometimes, learners sought their advice about family difficulties or even money troubles. "I still go to her for advice about personal things and work things," a former learner said. A frequent request was for guidance about the learners' career path. Another was for help coping with what one learner called "hospital systems issues," such as trouble getting through to a physician or arranging for a diagnostic test in a reasonable time frame. The attendings will generally be able to cut through the red tape and get the job done.

The 12 attendings do not simply make themselves available; they are also alert for situations in which they can proactively help out. At table rounds, they made sure to include extra material in their talks that would be of interest to particular team members. "I will be certain to mention visceral and cutaneous leishmaniasis," one of the attendings told us, "because they are endemic in the part of the world the intern is from." We heard another attending urging two medical students to view an interventional radiology procedure involving the abdomen because "GI is your thing." He also had a handout on the procedure he wanted to share with them.

A former learner recalled that when she was an intern, she was intensely worried about her lack of knowledge of intravenous catheters; she did not, for example, know the difference between a central line and a dialysis catheter. When she confessed her problem to her attending, she "sat me down and got out a catheter, and took something that I was especially concerned about and really made it easy for me."

At various points of the day, our attendings check in with the team, by text or in person, and they often make a late afternoon or nightly call to see if help is needed. If it's a hectic time, they may volunteer to talk with a patient's relatives or even temporarily take over a few patients so that a frazzled learner can complete his or her shift on time.

The attendings understand that a word of support or sympathy can often go a long way. A learner told us, for example, about one of his patients who was suffering with chronic pain and depression. The team had enlisted the help of the acute pain service, but suddenly the pain specialists signed off, saying they had done everything they could. "It put us in this position of, we're general medicine," the learner recalled. "What can *we* do?" The learner called her attending that night to provide an update and told her about the patient. " 'This sucks,' is basically what she said," the learner reported, "and she said, 'They put you in a bad situation and that's really frustrating. You're doing everything that you can.' And so it was nice. It was like she sort of reinforced what we were trying to do."

Our 12 attendings do identify with their learners and want the best for them, attitudes that their learners soon recognize and draw comfort from. This comment by one of the attendings makes the point:

> Oftentimes, I ask for July or August because I really love the newbies. I love when they're new and kind of excited. But I also feel really compelled to kind of set the stage, set expectations, help them kind of get a really good start on what it means to provide good inpatient care. Sometimes, if you don't get a good start right off the bat, then you kind of go down the other end. So, I feel a real responsibility.

The learners acknowledged feeling more engaged when they realized how much their attendings enjoyed teaching and how much these world-class physicians wanted to keep learning. "He's still just, you know, very enthusiastic about what he is teaching," a current learner told us, "and very curious, very much there to discover new things along with you." That frame of mind, universal among the 12 attendings, helped create a probing, intellectually stimulating climate that served both the team and patients well.

In pursuit of the best possible care for their patients, the attendings insisted that team members not automatically accept an attending's diagnostic or treatment proposals. If a learner had a different view, he or she was expected to challenge the attending.

We witnessed an exchange between a medical student and one of our attendings. When the attending disagreed with the learner's assessment of a patient's symptom, the learner responded, "Oh, O.K." The attending quickly responded, "Don't just melt away. I expect push-back." As another attending put it: "Stick to your guns. If you really hear it the way you heard it, make sure you don't give up on that." The goal is twofold: to foster independent thinking and to get the team members into the habit of advocating for their patients.

Such independent thinking is necessary, as our attendings are well aware, because they are fallible. They don't know all the answers. A former learner remembered an example:

> There have been times when he has asked question, question, question. Nobody knows, and then he admits that he doesn't know either. So everybody goes and looks it up. So it's that level of informality. The whole thing turns out to be a fun learning experience.

The attendings are also quick to admit their errors. "When I make a mistake, I tell them," one of the attendings reported. "I say, 'That's exactly what you don't want to do, is just what I did in there. Remember that. Don't ever do that.'" Each of the attendings had a store of personal mistakes that he or she would draw upon when relevant; they recognized that failure is the most valuable of teaching opportunities.

While rounding, we heard the following exchange between an attending and his team member:

INTERN: The patient's blood pressure has decreased since we started the medication.

ATTENDING: [High-fiving the senior resident] You were right! I said it wouldn't go down, but you said to wait and see and you were right. I owe you one.

The willingness of the attendings to admit ignorance or error had another important consequence. It contributed to the creation of a safe environment for learners by making mistakes a natural and inevitable aspect of the clinical learning process. If attendings have no hesitation about airing their limitations, it becomes much easier for learners to accept their own with a minimum of embarrassment.

The attendings have a variety of ways of getting that across to learners. Here's how one of them does it:

You don't have to "tolerate" things, you know. If there's something that I'm doing that's not helpful to you, I want you to tell me that now, not when we do mid-month feedback, because I'll adapt to what works for you. But you have to be comfortable enough to share that with me.

From their first encounters with a new team, the attendings clearly lay out their expectations as to the learners' responsibilities. Individual goals are set for the medical students, the interns, and the residents, including what they should get out of their weeks on the wards. The 12 attendings tend to set the bar high. A current learner described for us how his attending furthered those expectations:

You can tell you're being pushed to do what you're capable of, but you're being pushed with positivity and like, "Hey, I think you can do this for your patient. I think you're good enough to really take ownership and be the primary manager for this patient's care." It's a very supportive and positive way of getting you to put yourself out there and push yourself to your limits.

From a learner's perspective, the freedom to make independent patient-care decisions was probably the most important example of the attendings' support. That was only possible, of course, because of the layers of protection provided by the attending, the senior resident, and the consultants. This is where the rubber meets the road, where learners develop the clinical skills and the self-assurance to become practicing physicians. As one of the attendings tells her teams, "My job is to protect you from making a mistake that will wipe away your confidence."

A former learner recalled a moment when her attending urged her to take the lead in a difficult conversation with a patient. It was a challenging assignment, but the learner felt "completely comfortable," she said, "knowing that the attending was there in a supportive role if I had any kind of questions. And she really sat back and let me take the lead." The learner recognized that it might have been much easier for the attending to just have the conversation herself. "I'm toward the end of residency now," the learner said. "I'm realizing how valuable those experiences are in preparing me for future practice."

The time learners spend leading conversations or bedside presentations also serves to prepare them for another kind of future activity—as teachers, as attending physicians.

Our attendings generally give learners substantial leeway in their clinical decision-making. We heard of several instances in which the attending had one plan in mind while the learner proposed something different. If the learner's plan was not going to harm the patient or delay patient care, the attending approved its implementation.

A current learner spoke of his experience with one of the 12 attendings:

> I have had attendings where minor things like pain medicines or minor things like just doses of the same medicine, they would not want you to even experiment with doses. They want their dose and that's what they want. [Our current attending] was like, "Yeah, sure. You think that's going to work? Just do it. Try it. Make sure you have enough safeguards around that you won't end up killing the patient, but try it. And if it doesn't work, great. Come back to what I am saying or, if it works, even better! I will learn from you!"

We suspect that a key reason why our attendings felt comfortable admitting their own mistakes and allowing the team to have substantial autonomy in medical decision-making is that the attendings had true confidence in their own abilities. Insecurity often breeds micromanagement and bravado.

In the rare instances when the learner's plan fails, the attendings look for a way to move on without embarrassing the learner or destroying the learner's confidence and relationship with the patient. Here's an example as told to us by a current learner:

> At no point did she throw me under the bus or make the patient feel that way. I think she just sort of said, "We've done exactly what we said we were going to do. We discussed this plan of controlling your pain and now we're going to move to the alternative form of treatment which is what you want." And I think that made the patient happy, and it made me not feel like I was marginalized or disrespected in any way.

In that way, the attending made it possible for the learner to continue his management of the patient, and his education, in a positive frame of mind. Contrast that with the negative feelings of an errant learner who was embarrassed or even ridiculed in front of other team members. Learning flourishes best in a safe, supportive environment.

To that end, the 12 attending physicians strongly believe in positive feedback. Correction in the clinical setting, they believe, needs to be very different from that in a typical classroom. An attending explained: "I need to be able to tell them what they need to do better without them interpreting that as me giving them a grade."

Our attendings avoided the word "wrong" like the plague. Again and again, learners told us that the correction process is not judgmental, that it never feels demeaning or condescending. When a learner made a mistake, attendings engaged him or her in a discussion, often asking questions to find out what led to the incorrect conclusion. A former learner offered an extreme example: "You could say, 'I think this patient is sick because there was an alien invasion last night.' He would be, like, 'That's really a great idea, but what do you think about this?'"

There are all kinds of mistakes that a learner can make, of course, starting with the simple inability to answer a question. The 12 attendings generally started out with simple questions for the medical students on the team, geared to their knowledge level. If a learner seemed to be having difficulty with a question or came up with the wrong answer, the attendings generally redirected the question to another learner, with or without comment. A current learner told us about making a wrong suggestion and what his attending had to say about it:

> So he was like, "No, no, it's O.K. You probably said this because you figured this thing, which is a good thought process, but in this case it's not really applicable because of this thing." So that made me feel O.K. I wasn't as stupid as I might have sounded. So that is, I think, very, very important. I mean, it keeps you going.

When one of our attendings gives a learner feedback after a presentation and in front of other team members, the attending does so in a manner calculated to avoid upsetting the presenter. Here are some feedback samples we observed:

- Excellent presentation. Good job. But I want to talk about [the patient] medically. You didn't say this, but I saw in his chart that he had not been able to lie flat in two years.

- Excellent, you gave us all the essential stuff. You have to remember he came to us for chest discomfort, but you gave us too much on his psychiatric and family history. Write it in the medical record, but you can omit most of it for your oral presentation.

- Very well organized. Nice succinct story. Most remarkable was his systolic was 90. You mentioned stopping his fluids, but is his blood pressure back to normal?

If there was an error in patient care, our attendings' first reaction was to determine how and why it happened, what might have affected the learner's performance. A former learner described that kind of encounter:

> He would stop and say, "Just a second. What happened?" You know, before blaming him, saying, "Oh, that person is terrible. . ." And he gives so much credit to everyone, in terms of trying to understand what were the circumstances, why this happened.

In seeking to understand such an error, the attendings would call on their relationships with team members, looking for reasons in a learner's personal life. A former learner recalled that his attending would ask: "How are you? How's the wife? Everything O.K. at home?"

There are rare occasions when anger may surface. "I come down hard on them," one attending told us, "if the mistake they make is out of laziness or inattentiveness or not checking something. A couple of residents here have a very cavalier attitude, and that really frustrates me!"

Another attending was sorely tempted to vent when she looked over a learner's notes concerning a patient who had come in the night before with dizziness, which of course requires a full and complete history. Yet the learner's history of the patient read exactly like the emergency room note, and he told the same story in the same way on rounds. It wasn't the first time the learner had cut corners, and his attending walked him into the patient's room and they took the patient's history together. "We had a conversation," the attending told us, "and I said, 'I think you're a better physician than what you're showing me.'"

Far more evident than anger in the 12 attendings' behavior is their sense of humor, which serves as a key ingredient in relieving tensions and creating a safe and supportive environment (Figure 4.2). "Half of his communication is through humor," a current learner told us, "so it makes. . . rounding very comfortable." The humor tends to be self-deprecating, although it is sometimes aimed at the learners as well. "Because he is able to make fun of himself in front of us," another current learner added, "when he teases other people, it doesn't seem like it's done in a mean-spirited way."

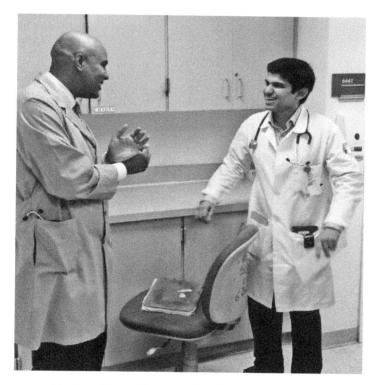

FIGURE 4.2 Attending and learner joking during rounds.

The jokes generally emerge out of a given situation as attending and team make their rounds. Here's one we watched develop. An attending spotted some writing on a patient's hand. "What's this?" he asked. "Something real important," the patient responded. "Oh," said the attending, "I thought you went clubbing last night."

Humor is a time-honored technique of establishing a rapport with people in general, and it also serves that function within a clinical team. We heard one of our attendings respond to an intern who suggested discharging a patient from the hospital: "Somebody could be dead, and you'd discharge them. He's ready to go. Don't worry about the smell." The attending and team members had a good laugh. In addition to being an example of joshing, the comment is a mild example of gallows humor, a traditional way physicians cope with the life-threatening and otherwise onerous circumstances they encounter daily. It can, however, be overdone. We will discuss the matter at greater length in Chapter 7.

In the next two chapters, we focus less on the people skills of the 12 attendings and more on their day-to-day teaching tools and techniques. The topics vary greatly, from the cure for a blank look to the uses of mnemonics and whiteboards, but they have a common origin in the practice of some awesome physician-teachers.

MAIN POINTS

1. The 12 attendings all created a safe and supportive learning environment but used various strategies to do so, such as supporting team members in both their professional and personal lives, being clear in their expectations of learners, seeking to understand errors rather than admonishing a learner, and using humor to stimulate learning.

2.   The attendings provide positive feedback and are completely engaged during rounds. They make themselves available to learners and are eager to help them. The attendings also get to know the learners on a personal level in order to build trusting relationships with their teams.

3.   The attendings admit their own mistakes and welcome challenges from learners, demonstrating their conviction that a mistake is a prime learning experience. Learners engage in clinical decision-making knowing that their attending will support and protect them in case of an oversight.

Further Reading

Hewson, M. G., & Little, M. L. (1998). Giving feedback in medical education. *Journal of General Internal Medicine, 13*(2), 111–116.

In this article, the authors sought to validate the feedback recommendations found in the medical education literature and to provide additional insight into these recommendations. Participants in a faculty development course for improving the teaching of the medical interview provided narratives of their own feedback experiences, including what they found to be helpful and unhelpful. The authors found that effective feedback techniques included creating nonthreatening learning environments, asking for others' thoughts before giving feedback, being nonjudgmental, and offering suggestions for improvement.

Ziegler, J. B. (1998). Use of humour in medical teaching. *Medical Teacher, 20*(4), 341–348.

Although the use of humor in medical teaching is thought to be widespread, little is known about its potential value in the learning environment. What the few studies that have been done found is that use of humor can reduce anxiety, build confidence, and even encourage diverse thinking. However, even though it appears it may enhance the educational experience, humor has not been well-researched.

Martinez, W., Hickson, G. B., Miller, B. M., Doukas, D. J., Buckley, J. D., Song, J. . . . Lehmann, L. S. (2014). Role-modeling and medical error disclosure: A national survey of trainees. *Academic Medicine, 89*(3), 482–489.

The authors of this article examined the association between positive and negative role-modeling and trainees' attitudes and behaviors regarding medical error disclosure. They found that trainees overall reported more frequent exposure to positive role-modeling. However, more frequent exposure to negative role-modeling was associated with an increased likelihood of nondisclosure in response to a harmful error. Thus, the act of role modeling should be considered an important element in organizational safety culture.

5

Bedside and Beyond

■□■

The good physician treats the disease; the great physician treats the patient who has the disease.

—WILLIAM OSLER

AS THE PRACTICE of medicine has become increasingly complex over the years, the clinical education of medical students has inevitably become ever more complicated and demanding. There is so much new information to be conveyed, so many new treatments, so many more challenging inpatients, so much new technology. At the same time, learners' hours on the job have been substantially reduced. These developments have whittled away at a centuries-old, essential aspect of clinical education: bedside teaching.

Well before the 2003 change in interns' hours, concerns were being raised over how little time learners were engaged in direct patient interaction; studies suggested that less than 25% of clinical teaching was taking place at the bedside.[1] But, by 2013, a team from Johns Hopkins discovered interns were examining and conversing with patients just 12% of the time. More than 40% of their workday was spent at a computer.[2]

The invasion of technology, an attending physician has written,[3] has led to "the surrender of bedside diagnostic acumen and a generation of doctors with strikingly redundant clinical abilities and poor diagnostic concepts." He concluded: "If I were to suffer a medical problem, I would prefer to be seen by a grey-haired doctor with his beloved stethoscope and hyperpigmented digits (the result of repeated percussion), rather than a young one surrounded by flashing screens and noisy machines."

Although their views may not be so extreme, the 12 outstanding attending physicians we observed and interviewed are well aware of the pressures that are pulling learners away from the bedside. They don't like it. They are strong supporters and insistent practitioners of bedside teaching, determined to give their learners as much of it as possible. One of the attendings told us, "As we move toward shorter rounds and shorter time for our learners, more of the time we've been spending in [table] rounds and presenting has to be spent with the patient and the problem."

The 12 attendings have found ways to adjust their schedules to the peaks and valleys of their learners' days. "She knew that there didn't have to be an hour of teaching every day if we were too busy," a current learner said of his attending. She also won the gratitude of her residents by having medical students do abbreviated presentations on team rounds, saving residents precious minutes for their other work. "I really appreciated that!" one of her residents exclaimed. (The attending would listen to the medical students' full presentations at one-on-one meetings.)

What could abbreviated presentations during rounds look like? The traditional presentation on rounds is the "E-SOAP" presentation, which stands for Events, Subjective, Objective, Assessment, and Plan. It includes having the learner present the events from overnight, subjective complaints the patient may be having, objective findings on the physical exam beginning with the vital signs, relaying all of the test and other results from the previous day, and concluding with the assessment and plan. To make rounds more efficient, some attendings may choose to focus on just the events overnight and assessment and plan by problem (so-called "EAP" presentations). If the patient had a fever overnight, that would be listed as a problem to discuss. The same goes for a low sodium or continued abdominal pain or new-onset diarrhea.

Another attending will show up at the team room on an afternoon to do teaching targeted at third-year students and will inform them he wants their undivided attention. On the other hand, he tells the interns and residents in the room—most of whom are on the computer—that he only wants half *their* attention. "It's just hard for busy residents and interns to say, 'O.K., I can give you my undivided attention for the next 20 minutes,'" he said.

One of the attendings reported: "I round on every patient every day, but I don't round on every patient with the team every day." That kind of arrangement, he said, allows them to give their full attention to the bedside rounds because it limits the team rounding time to two hours a day and they do not have to worry about, as he put it, "Oh, my God! Am I ever going to get to put an order in?"

A current learner told us of another accommodation made by one of the attendings. "If we don't see my patients as a [team]," the learner said, "he will come back and see them individually with me. I've never had anyone do that before." Most of the attendings made it a point to see every patient assigned to their team every day whether they were newly admitted patients or existing ones.

As you might expect, the attendings are excellent bedside teachers. To begin with, they are virtuoso clinicians and diagnosticians.

A former learner acknowledged that his method of conducting an abdominal exam was learned from one of our 12 attendings at a patient's bedside. The patient had a known abdominal mass, and the attending was palpating the abdomen. "I was like, wow, that is very different from how I've been doing it," the former learner recalled, "but now I'll do it his way."

Another former learner described his attending: "His physical exam skills were amazing. He would often pick up on things just by looking at the patients. When he would notice something about the patient that maybe was unrelated to the patient's main complaint, he would use it as a teaching point."

In one instance, we saw an attending in the process of examining a patient hospitalized for a different reason point out a series of yellow globules on a patient's chest, indicative of damage from sun exposure. When his team of learners was in the room of a patient with cyclic vomiting, that same attending had them examine the patient's teeth, even though the patient had not complained of any dental problems. The attending knew they would find damage caused by stomach acid.

Our attendings share many attributes and attitudes. When we asked them to identify the primary goal of bedside teaching, for example, their answers were remarkably similar. "Providing not just random trivial facts," one replied, "but patient-applicable knowledge [that learners] can carry forward, taking it to the bedside of the next patient and figuring where it fits and where it doesn't fit."

Another attending spoke of learners applying this knowledge "to make a good clinical decision," while a third cited the need to present the knowledge "in a way that people can remember."

The 12 attendings do have their individual instructional strategies and tactics, however. In this chapter, we discuss some of the many and various ways in which they go about their inspired teaching.

It may seem like the most basic and elementary of lessons an attending can teach his or her learners: If you want to find out what's wrong with a patient, ask the patient. One form of such inquiry is the physical examination. Whether it's performed by a learner or an attending, the exam needs to be deliberate and thorough, with the fingers asking and answering questions about the patient's condition. The more obvious form of questioning is verbal: talk to the patient about his or her symptoms and feelings.

The problem-oriented medical interview is a staple of traditional medical practice, but the invasion of new technologies and the ramped-up time pressures on attendings and learners have sometimes diluted the clinical focus on the patient. A former learner described how his attending combats that trend: "Instead of just looking at what we know from lab studies or imaging or talking to consultants, he often asks patients what they first noticed when they were diagnosed with the condition. . .back to the original complaint."

A current learner spoke of his attending's insistence on individualizing patient care. "A lot of times," he said, "attendings don't kind of talk to the patient as much. We don't kind of look at the whole situation of the patient when we make decisions. He does."

Patients generally enter a hospital because of a single acute problem. "On a busy call day," a former learner told us, "we kind of tunnel our vision on this one big thing. But if you talk with the patients, there might be several other sub-acute or chronic problems. If there was anything significant going on with a patient, [our attending] required us to be on top of that. And it's not that it took a lot more time or energy to provide more holistic care for the patient instead of just focusing on one thing."

One of the hallmarks of the 12 attendings is the thoroughness with which they approach both patient care and their teaching responsibilities. A former learner recalled an extreme example of that dedication, a visit he made to a patient with his attending and nine other learners.

The attending wanted the learners to listen to the patient's lungs as the patient said "Eeee."[4] His attending, the former learner said, was not one of those teachers who would do the test himself and say, "Oh, he's got a good Murphy's sign," and then tell the team members to come back and do the test on their own time, knowing that most of them would never make it back.

This attending insisted that every member of the team, one after the other, put their stethoscopes to the patient's chest while the patient pronounced the "Eeeeee." "We stood there," the former learner said, "the whole team. It must have taken 20 minutes, you know, with the attending apologizing to the patient, being nice to the patient. It was kind of funny, and the patient was laughing by the end of it, but that was how he did it. He was very thorough."

While making rounds with one of the 12 attendings, we saw two examples within an hour of his intense attention to his patients and his automatic sharing of his findings with his learners. The exchanges occurred after the team left the patients' rooms.

> ATTENDING: Time to critique the attending. Why did I question her about depression?
>
> INTERN: Because she started tearing up.
>
> ATTENDING: She said, "I feel bad." There's often a little window you get in the course of a conversation. The key is to follow that window. It's important to think about picking up and following those cues.

A short time later, another patient, another insight. The attending addresses the medical student.

> ATTENDING: So there was something we heard when we were leaving the bedside.
>
> MEDICAL STUDENT: Something about anxiety.
>
> ATTENDING [TO INTERN]: That's something we should make her PCP [primary care provider] aware of.

Inevitably, with a group of people examining patients, there will be differences of opinion. One of the 12 attendings told us how he handles that situation. "We're going to listen together, look together, feel together," he said, "and I discipline myself to ask the learner, 'What did you hear, what did you see, what did you feel?' before I say anything."

The attending gave an example of a resident who said, "I think that's a diastolic murmur." The attending was confident it was systolic, but he did not say so directly so as not to undermine the resident's confidence. Instead, he told her,

"Maybe I got this wrong. Let me listen again." And he taught her the technique of listening and, at the same time, matching the murmur to the pulse. "Then I didn't have to do anything more," the attending said. "She was able to say, 'Oh, yeah, that's systolic.'"

He described how an exam disagreement with a learner should proceed:

> If we're in agreement, that's great; if we're not in agreement, then I re-examine with the learner. If we're still not in agreement, I say, 'Let's listen right here and listen very specifically for this or let's feel right here and what do you feel now?' If that doesn't work, then we're going to have to come back in the afternoon.

On patient rounds, one of the 12 attendings told us, she follows an "on-the-fly" teaching style. "It depends on what comes up on a day-to-day basis," she said. "So like, when we first saw the woman with the traumatic brain injury, we walk in and she's got the sand bed and so we talk about mattress choices, about turning schedules, about sacral decubitus ulcers. If somebody has a catheter, it's let's (a) take it out and (b) talk about catheter-related UTIs."

But spontaneity is just one aspect of our attendings' conduct of patient rounds. To begin with, they have examined the patients and read their charts before the rounds ever take place (Figure 5.1). Based on what they have learned and their knowledge of their team of learners, the attendings conjure up relevant teaching points and clarifications in advance. So patient rounds are actually a combination of attendings' impromptu insights inspired by the events of the particular patient encounter and their calculated lessons.

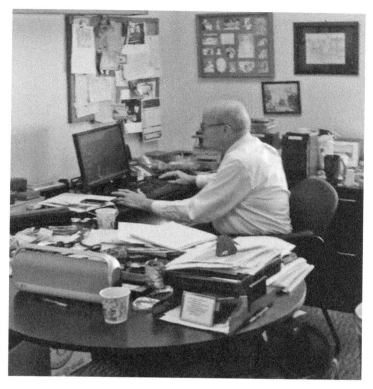

FIGURE 5.1 Attending reading over a patient's record.

The "on-the-fly" attending, for example, presided over the following exchange after a medical student presented on a patient:

MEDICAL STUDENT: We checked his lactates.

ATTENDING: We can check his lactates until the cows come home. What are we doing to him now?

MEDICAL STUDENT: Could we send him home with his medication?

RESIDENT: That's a good idea if he was dying to go home. I think we risk nonadherence with him.

ATTENDING: I would worry that he would not want to come back.

MEDICAL STUDENT: He asked about the biopsy. I told him I would defer to the team, but it would probably be through the mouth or skin.

ATTENDING: Good, good.

MEDICAL STUDENT: So we should continue with LR [lactated ringers solution]?

ATTENDING: I'm going to make my LR face. [She turns to the resident.] There's a paper on my desk, and we're going to do a point-counterpoint about using LR.

RESIDENT: I'm not defending it.

ATTENDING: But you will be. [She addresses the team as a whole.] When we come out of the patient's room, someone tell me: What's a fever?

The exchange initially appears to be simply an example of impromptu instruction. But it turns out the attending has anticipated the reference to LR and has already planned a later, more detailed discussion of the topic.

In fact, by their very nature, patient rounds are not the ideal setting for the delivery of a full-scale teaching script on a particular symptom or disease. It steals too much time from the already limited time available for patient rounds. Instead, our attendings seek to anticipate teaching moments and prepare brief lessons that are relevant to the patients who will be seen on rounds.

"Some attendings," a current learner complained, "go on and on about things that aren't related to the patient, or they'll just talk too long. And once that happens, you start to space out and zone out." On the other hand, his attending, one of our outstanding 12, is "really good at finding teaching points, little pearls."

The attendings especially like to scope out learner confusions or errors ahead of time so they can take full advantage of these prized teaching moments—nothing like a mistake, yours or others', to fix a lesson in the memory. One attending told us he can anticipate where his learners will be "stuck" with about 70% of the patients. For 10% of the patients, he added, "I will be stuck myself at the start and have to try to figure out what's going on." Another attending added: "I am always ahead of the house staff, though I may not let them know it. I feel most comfortable that way, anticipating and then giving them the space to catch up." That kind of preparation was nearly universal among the 12 attendings.

An attending gave us the backstory for a teaching moment we had witnessed earlier. He had seen the patient and gone over the notes a learner had prepared, and he was confident that the learner had missed a significant symptom. "So I kind of went into that room," he said, "knowing we may find something here that's different from what I've read going in." Later, in the hallway, the learner and the other members of the team benefitted from the attending's insight. "It helps them pay attention at the bedside," he said. "Much of what I've learned about interviewing patients I've learned from watching other people do it."

Some of the attendings are silent observers while learners conduct bedside rounds, speaking only when there is an issue that needs immediate clarification, otherwise holding their comments until the team leaves the patient's room.

Several of the attendings, though, tend to be more vocal, directing the interaction with the patient and occasionally offering suggestions and corrections during the bedside presentation. We saw that happen when a medical student asked the patient, "How do you feel about going home today?" The attending interrupted: "No, no. Tell him what the plan is for the day." In the hallway, the attending explained that the patient might have kicked up a fuss about leaving. Better to say that the medical team was recommending that the patient go home that day.

The attendings save their most intense and detailed post-bedside feedback for the senior resident, who is the team leader. Here's how an attending characterizes his daily critique, delivered via email:

> I fundamentally hold her responsible. Did you call a consult or not? Did you guys overdose or underdose this antibiotic? You asked this question and it was an awkward moment. If you had just asked this person first, it could have been a much smoother interaction. We were in that room too long. We boxed out the nurse when we were at bedside.

And here's the senior resident's characterization of the attending's feedback:

> Every afternoon after rounds, I get an email from him with a PDF of his notes from morning rounds. It really is step-by-step, what I said, what I should have said, what my body position was, whether something was good or what I could improve upon. It's extremely helpful because a lot of my actions on rounds are subconscious and I don't realize that I am doing it.

The 12 attendings work hard at tailoring their teaching to the disparate needs of the individual team members, whether at the bedside or during table rounds. It's not a simple task. Medical students, interns, and residents are by definition at different stages of their medical education and experience. And within each category, the learners have varied backgrounds and specialty interests.

"I get here early to look over all my patients," one of the attendings told us, "so I already know what the team should be telling me, and I already know what I want to teach them." He always has one simple teaching point to make and one higher level point. For instance, he said, "A patient is on subcutaneous heparin, scheduled for surgery the next morning, and I will ask, 'How soon do we need to stop the heparin?' After that, I'll move on to something more involved, I'll say, 'Now, let's go to subcutaneous Lovenox.'"

A former learner said his attending taught "to every level of learner," offering this example: "She would start out talking about the lab abnormalities when a liver is not functioning well, which is practical information no matter what specialty a learner is interested in. But then she would get into our patient's cirrhosis and the details of how to manage it."

Given the different educational levels in a team, though, there will always be moments when one or another learner just doesn't get it, doesn't understand some aspect of an attending's explanation. The 12 attendings keep an eye out for what one of them called "that blank look." She added: "I try to talk through processes out loud as much as possible because I think sometimes we jump from Point A to Point C and we skip Point B in the middle." That jump can easily cause the blank look to appear on learners' faces. When that happens, the attending said, "I just let it go, and go back to the learner later. And I go through the material again with him until he says, 'O.K. Now it makes sense.' We can't leave them with these big open gaps in the knowledge they need to take to the next patient."

Our attendings provide learners with a maximum of individual attention. At these sessions, the learners are encouraged to report any uncertainty about the material being covered. (Some attendings, at the start of a rotation, urge learners to keep a written list of items they're uncertain about for later discussion with the attendings.)

In addition to clarifying concepts and giving learners feedback, attendings use one-on-one meetings to ask learners for ideas to improve their own teaching. "I tell them I'm trying to get better every day, too," an attending said, "and so what can I do differently that would help you learn better? I had a senior resident who told me I was being too hard on the interns. That's fine! I found ways to build them up."

Another attending offers an unusual individual service for the medical student members of his team. He has them print paper copies of their notes. "I'll get out a red pen, just for fun," the attending said, "and I'll put on this frowny face, and I'll mark up their H & Ps and tell them to go back over them." It takes 10 minutes each, a strain on the attending's schedule, but he knows how valuable it is for learners. "If someone had done that for me," he said, "I would have been in a lot better shape. I had no idea how to do a note."

On patient rounds or on table rounds, the 12 attendings have their own distinctive styles of teaching (Figure 5.2). Some will deliver a five-minute discourse in the hallway after seeing a patient because the topic is so spot-on to the patient's main complaint. Others are more inclined to save their lectures for table rounds. But all of the attendings have at their mental beck and call dozens of *teaching scripts*, short lectures that deal with particular diseases or findings—an approach to hyponatremia, for example. Their mastery of the scripts gives the attendings the ability to vary the length of their presentation depending upon the venue—shorter at bedside, longer at table rounds.

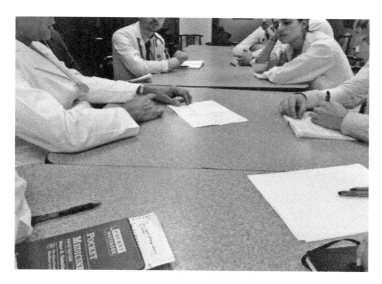

FIGURE 5.2 Table rounds with the team.

According to their learners, current and former, the attendings deliver "high-yield" lectures. "I think he understands really well kind of where we are coming from," a current learner said of his attending. "He can teach us a whole humongous topic in 15 minutes, and we all, in the end, probably have a better understanding than if we sat down with a textbook for three hours. That's happened multiple times this week already."

In addition to their presentations on bedside and table rounds, some of the attendings will, once or twice a week, gather the medical students on their teams for a brief lecture, usually no more than 10 minutes, geared to their comprehension level (Figure 5.3). "That's one thing I took away from him," a former student said. "Now I do these clinical pearl talks too, like from aortic stenosis to central line-associated bloodstream infections."

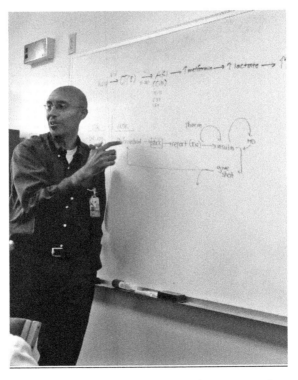

FIGURE 5.3 Attending conducting a short teaching session after rounds.

The 12 attendings look for ways to pique the learners' interest in their lectures, beyond the learners' inherent interest in getting smart about their chosen profession. They will often use a joke or a topical reference as a way to firm the contents of their lectures in the learners' memories.

We saw the following table rounds exchange after an intern presented on a patient who had an unexplained stroke:

INTERN: I'm thinking DVT [deep vein thrombosis] and getting an ultrasound. [The intern was concerned about a paradoxical embolism due to a heart defect.]

ATTENDING: I think that's perfect. In terms of diagnosing, let's say it is negative.

INTERN: I'm not entirely certain. . . .

ATTENDING: It's controversial. The opinions wax and wane. Are you guys football fans?

At that point, the attending pulled several copies of an article from his pocket and handed them around. It was about the New England Patriots defensive star, Tedy Bruschi, who suffered a mild stroke shortly after playing in the 2005 Pro Bowl. He had a patent foramen ovale and was partially paralyzed. After eight months of rehabilitation, he was back on the field.

ATTENDING: Look it over and tell me what you think.. . . In terms of atrial fib, do you feel good about ruling that out as a cause?

INTERN: I think so.

ATTENDING: So, here's another [important] article. It definitely changed the way I do things. I read this article and was convinced that getting 30-day event monitors is the right thing to do.

The attending then distributed a 2014 article from the *New England Journal of Medicine* that found that 30 days of noninvasive ambulatory electrocardiogram (ECG) monitoring improved the detection of atrial fibrillation five-fold compared with standard short-duration ECG monitoring.[5]

Bringing paper copies of articles to table rounds can be cumbersome, but it does make it much more likely that the team will look through the paper and learn from it.

The 12 attendings have different ways of providing extra reading material. A current learner described how his attending goes about it. "If we've been talking about antibiotic coverage or something and it comes up during patient rounds," he told us, "she'll hop onto the computer right there and pull things up and show them to you. Or she'll forward us papers, like right after rounds. If you like evidence-based medicine, it's nice to see that." Nor does the attending forget that she sent the material. "The next time the same problem appears," the learner said, "she'll be like: 'So did you read those guidelines we talked about?'"

Most attending physicians, a former learner told us, won't bother to explain medical school-level material, telling team members to just look it up. "Look it up is O.K.," he said, "but you are so busy.. . ." His attending "looks it up *with* you. He forces you to spend the time doing the research, because of which you remember things."

The 12 attendings are alert to topics that may go uncovered. For example, one of the attendings lectures on billing, and another of our attendings gave his team a list of nursing homes he has found to be reliable. "I don't think any residency does a really good job of preparing residents for the transition to being a faculty member," she said.

We close this chapter with a potpourri of teaching ideas and techniques our attendings use:

- The memorized teaching scripts are a staple of a medical educator's tool kit, developed and refined over years. Several of the attendings shared their scripts with the learners. As one said, "They can do whatever they want with them, ignore it, modify it, adapt it to your needs."

- "I have long believed that learners like the people who are teaching them to be *smart*," one of our attendings said. "So for the first few sessions in a month, I try to show overwhelming knowledge of medicine to dazzle a little." It also, he added, suggests to learners that these "dazzling things are a part of their future."

- When a team orders a test, there is an assumption that the result will be positive. "I always say," an attending told us, "presume it is negative so that whatever happens, you can go to the next step. Otherwise, if it doesn't show anything, you are all going to be sitting there in the same spot."

- A popular device among attending physicians in general—and for our 12 as well—is the *mnemonic*, a word whose letters typically represent a medical grouping such as the names of the bones in the hand or the symptoms of a disease.[6] For example, a classic mnemonic for recalling the indications for acute hemodialysis is "A-E-I-O-U."

- One attending carried a whiteboard about with him, using it to take notes—lab values during rounds, for example—or to sketch parts of the body during a table rounds lecture or a bedside talk. A current learner compared his attending's sketches to looking at a PowerPoint presentation on a screen: "It's complete night and day in terms of being able to follow along and pay attention and be invested in what's being taught." (Other attendings use index cards to the same effect.)

- Another attending plays a game called "Around the World." If he has a question that has five or six right answers, he calls on each team member to give one answer, starting with the medical students. Saying "I don't know" is allowed. "I have to play, too," the attending said, "and if it gets to me a second time, it's really hard."

- Learners and attendings are under greater pressure these days than in the past. One of the attendings has responded by creating what he calls the Box of Unprofessionalism. In this room, he and his learners occasionally gather to joke, cuss, and generally vent about what's bothering them. The only rule: They must continue to be respectful of one another.

A current learner of one of the 12 attendings summed up much of what we have written about in this chapter: "The most important thing wasn't getting out on time or showing you knew more than anybody else. The most important thing was to be with the patient at the bedside, caring for them and their families. That's why you were there and that's why you were a doctor."

In the following chapter, we consider a significant aspect of clinical education—the attending's thought process and how it is applied and shared with his or her learners. Among other matters, we explore the Socratic method of questioning and the value of second thoughts.

MAIN POINTS

1. The attendings made bedside teaching (or the teaching that occurs just outside of a patient's room) a mainstay of their approach. They felt that the best way to learn was from the patients themselves. They combined their physical examination and questioning of the patient with the presentation of relevant teaching points.

2. Attendings taught that information learned from a current patient should be applied to the next patient. In this way, what is taught builds on itself, creating a solid foundation of knowledge.

3. Attendings would not only teach to the team but also would be alert to any need to provide individual instruction. They recognized that team members have different learning capacities and sought to prevent knowledge gaps from developing in every level of learner.

Further Reading

Peters, M., & ten Cate, O. (2014). Bedside teaching in medical education: A literature review. *Perspectives on Medical Education*, 3(2), 76–88.

In this article, the authors conducted a literature review on the use of bedside teaching in medical education. Although bedside teaching was once the primary modality for teaching clinical skills, its use has declined in recent years. Thus, the authors sought to determine bedside teaching's role and strengths in teaching clinical skills and why its use has declined. The authors found that trainees and patients alike seem to value bedside teaching. But, because of shortened admittance of patients and an increased reliance on technology to determine diagnosis, bedside teaching is on the decline.

Irby, D. M. (1994). Three exemplary models of case-based teaching. *Academic Medicine*, 69(12), 947–953.

In this article, Irby describes three distinctive ways of organizing teaching rounds: (1) case-bedside teaching, (2) case-lecture teaching and, (3) case-iterative teaching. These three models of teaching share five common characteristics including anchoring instruction in cases, actively involving learners in the process of teaching, modeling professional thinking and action, providing direction and feedback, and creating collaborative learning environments. Incorporating these five characteristics into the teaching process will facilitate the learning process.

McMahon, G. T., Marina, O., Kritek, P. A., & Katz, J. T. (2005). Effect of a physical examination teaching program on the behavior of medical residents. *Journal of General Internal Medicine*, 20(8), 710–714.

Although the physical exam is a critical component of determining diagnosis, its use as a diagnostic aid has declined. Thus, this study conducted a series of educational workshops for medical residents to determine whether such a program could increase the use of the physical examination among medical residents. After the program, there was a marked improvement in performance of the physical exam on rounds, and residents reported that their exam skills improved, as did their ability to teach these skills.

Ramani, S. (2008). Twelve tips for excellent physical examination teaching. *Medical Teacher*, 30(9–10), 851–856.

In this article, Ramani describes the key challenges in teaching the physical exam and offers 12 practical strategies that institutions and educators can use to promote high-quality physical examination teaching. The author describes the importance of the physical examination as it relates to patient–physician interactions and its role in the clinical diagnosis process.

6

How to Think About Thinking

■□■

The wise man doesn't give the right answers; he poses the right questions.

—CLAUDE LEVI-STRAUSS

ONE CURRENT LEARNER told us that he was mystified. "I don't know how she does it," he said of his attending physician, "but she teaches you without *teaching* you."

By the time many learners start their clinical rotations, they have spent years with teachers who provided them, in person and through readings, with all the required information. The students were expected to listen, read, and memorize for the final exam.

Our 12 outstanding attending physicians have a very different teaching style. "I approach it as more of a dialogue than a teaching," one of them told us. "I often just sort of make them teach themselves." Another attending added: "I stimulate them to think and work through the problems as opposed to me just telling them the answer."

In the team approach to clinical education, senior members oversee the learning experiences of junior members while attendings monitor patients' care and learners' progress. They also look for potential teaching moments, typically some kind of error or misunderstanding, to lead learners beyond "how" questions about a patient's ailments toward "why" questions. The goal: to help learners develop both the analytic and the intuitive components of clinical reasoning, the sine qua non of medical practice.

In this chapter, we describe how the 12 attendings go about that task—in essence, how they think about thinking and teach without teaching. We will explore the ways they develop their questions, share their own thought processes, and implant a desire for lifelong learning in their team members.

Clinical reasoning is the means by which seasoned physicians correctly diagnose patients' problems and develop appropriate treatments. It has two main components. The first is the ability to mentally stockpile and integrate information gathered in the process of treating vast numbers of patients and reading vast quantities of research studies. Physicians thereby learn to recognize patterns of clinical data, and that sometimes makes it possible for them to make instant, automatic diagnoses. The process is intuitive and nonanalytical.

The second major facet of physicians' clinical reasoning is analytical. Physicians painstakingly examine and weigh all the evidence, including a clinical history and physical examination of the patient. Hypotheses are developed, tested, and retested on the path toward differential diagnosis and a management plan.

Although quite different, the two components of clinical reasoning are complementary. In most cases, both analytical and nonanalytical elements play a role in the eventual decision. Studies have shown that an overreliance on the intuitive leap to diagnosis can lead to error.[1]

Clinical education has always tilted toward the analytical component of clinical reasoning. Learners spend their days examining patients and weighing differential diagnoses in terms of their probability. But many attendings, including our 12, also acknowledge in their teaching the intuitive aspects of clinical care.[2]

"Moving from intern to resident," one of the 12 told us, "gives you the ability to determine when a patient is sick or not. You have seen the spectrum of sick to not sick; you have processed thousands of pieces of information. Then, wow, something's different about a patient. And when you decide [to call a rapid response team], it's a visceral, gut feeling, and you have to trust yourself."

Another of our attendings said that he teaches using the questions he asks himself when he considers a patient, questions that sometimes cast doubt on accepted recommendations. "Where the questions come from I don't know," he continued. "Sometimes it's just a vision: Well, this is odd. Why is this? It might lead to nothing or it could be something."

In fact, questions are the essential tool that the 12 attendings use to explore the level of their learners' comprehension and to guide their learners' thinking and thought processes. Questions reveal learning opportunities.

"If a question comes to me," a current learner told us, "there's a reason it comes to me. I never feel that the attending is trying to put me in a place where I won't know the answer to the question. I think he's trying to assay the frontier of my knowledge. And I think the question is based on patients that I've seen recently so it's not completely out of the blue."

The attendings' questions serve another purpose: They inspire the *modest* degree of anxiety that makes learners more receptive to learning. Note the emphasis on "modest." As indicated in earlier chapters, our attendings go to great lengths to create a supportive, noncompetitive team environment for learners that minimizes insecurity and anxiety.[3] But our attendings also realize that complacency undermines learning and breeds poor patient care. Indeed, one way of thinking about how some attendings approach learning is to consider the relationship between learning and stress as depicted in Figure 6.1. This inverted U-shaped relationship indicates that learning is compromised with too little and too much anxiety. Finding that right amount of stress to induce in the learners is what attendings seek.

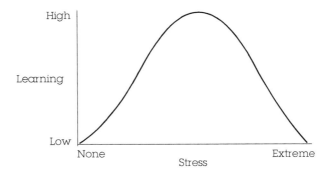

FIGURE 6.1 Learning-stress curve.

Most of the attendings' queries ask learners what conclusions they have reached about their patients as to diagnosis and treatment. Sometimes, a single exchange will suffice: "What dose would you give?" "When would you restart the med?" At other times, attendings will take a learner through a lengthy series of questions that carry the learner from a diagnosis to a treatment plan. All along the way, the attendings are probing to determine the level of the learners' understanding of the patient's condition. Here was an interaction between one of our attendings and a medical student discussing a patient with likely malabsorption:

ATTENDING: That's great, you discovered a new finding with this low calcium level. What did you want to do about it?

MEDICAL STUDENT: I'm not sure.

ATTENDING: O.K. Should we do any other diagnostic tests?

MEDICAL STUDENT: Maybe repeat the colonoscopy.

ATTENDING: Let's say the colonoscopy is negative. Would you do a study of the upper GI tract?

MEDICAL STUDENT: Probably.

ATTENDING: I agree with you. Patient's anemia may be related to malabsorption. We could do more blood tests or just start him on vitamin supplements. I'm not sure we need to do a vitamin blood test. Can we just start the supplements? Are you comfortable with that recommendation?

MEDICAL STUDENT: Yes.

ATTENDING: Why don't we talk to pharmacy about what's the best iron supplement to put through an IV. Where do you think you would start the dose at?

MEDICAL STUDENT: 2,000 milligrams

ATTENDING: That would be good if he wasn't starting out so low. He would never catch up. What we want to do is to give him more to get caught up and then go to maintenance. Are you O.K. with that plan?

MEDICAL STUDENT: Yes.

In their probings, the 12 attendings frequently employ hypotheticals, what-if scenarios, to spur learners to think outside their comfort zone. In the preceding exchange, for example, the attending asks, "What if the colonoscopy test results are negative?" Tests are often ordered on the expectation that they will produce positives, demonstrating the validity of a diagnosis. The what-if question requires learners to consider the impact of a negative result on their whole mental picture of the patient.

Along with hypotheticals, the attendings' questions often raise alternatives to the existing diagnosis or treatment plan, another challenge that forces learners to come up with a different way of thinking about the patient.

Hypotheticals and alternatives put learners in a circumstance that they are likely to face as practicing physicians, in which their conclusions are challenged, and they are forced to rethink them on their feet, in the middle of the action, with no time for preparation. These scenarios can also trigger discussions that move learners beyond the specific patient toward higher level topics.

Another kind of question our attendings sometimes use might be called a non-question question. It is asked not so much to elicit information as to inspire second thoughts. Two current learners recalled an example:

> FIRST LEARNER: A lot of times, when he says, "Oh, did that guy get a CT scan?" Whether I do or don't recall ordering the test, it makes me second-guess myself. I double-check my work. It makes you go back and review and really know your patients better.

> SECOND LEARNER: When he asked about the CT scan, I think he knew that it wasn't done, you know, but it made them question, "Does the patient need a CT scan?"

> FIRST LEARNER: That may be just his way of asking us, you know, did we really complete our workup? His

nice way of saying, "Did we do everything we should have for this patient?"

The most challenging type of questioning our attending physicians pursue is rooted in the so-called Socratic method, credited to the ancient Greek philosopher, Socrates. Legend has it that Socrates thought it no accident that his mother was a midwife because his teaching technique helped students give birth to new ideas.[4]

The technique calls for the teacher to ask a student a series of linked questions, each question built on the previous answer, thus leading to the self-discovery of a truth that had existed, unrecognized, in the student's brain. Teaching, as it were, without teaching.

Socratic questions leveled by the 12 attendings are not intended to determine learners' knowledge level. The attendings already know that; they routinely diagnose their learners as well as their patients. So, as the questions move in a logical sequence from one concept to the next, the learners can intuitively respond to the attendings' questions all the way to their conclusion. The goal is to guide the learners to a new, higher level of understanding.

A current learner told us his experience with the Socratic method:

> They gauge where your knowledge is and then sort of put themselves in your brain and lead you down the path. They don't start the questions at a higher level such that you would be like, I just don't know that. Instead, they start slowly and they sort of leave a trail of bread crumbs for you to follow so that you're making connections all along the way. And you come out of that conversation feeling good because you came to the right place in the end.

The attendings' emphasis is always on learners' thought processes rather than the details of their work. There is no way learners can memorize all the facts involved in practicing medicine. What they can and must master are the methods, the ways of thinking that enable physicians to cope with their everyday challenges.

"Rather than feeding us factual information," a current learner said of his attending, "he teaches us the heuristics of medicine, how to approach a problem, so that we have a framework for going about it." That included learning to synthesize the key aspects of a patient's condition, to identify the "major points, the big decisions."

When an error occurs, the attendings delve into the learner's mental processes. A current learner described the approach: "If we propose the wrong plan, he will ask us to go through our reasoning process. So we will explain what we saw or thought that contributed to the wrong plan. Then he will explain maybe what we should have seen or thought, but he will certainly be very polite about it."

Learners' critical thinking is not, the 12 attendings insist, supposed to stop once a better plan is conceived. Learners are urged to constantly rethink their conclusions, reassess their priorities. We often heard the attendings say, "Looking back to last night, what else could you have done?" or something similar. They also, as part of the second-thought mandate, want their learners to ask them questions. The attendings want to be challenged. "When we can successfully stimulate our students to ask their own questions," says a professor in a study of college teaching, "we are laying the foundation for learning." [5] As a former learner stated when asked about one of the 12 attendings: "You can very easily disagree with him and challenge him, say that no, that's not the case. . .you can say whatever you think or you can say that you disagree."

There will always be patients who present new and different problems. There will always be new research results and medications and treatments to integrate into physicians' knowledge base and practice. To cope with such challenges, physicians will need to maintain that ability to think about thinking that they gained on their clinical rounds.

A current learner recalled hearing a speech by one of our 12 attendings:

> He talked about how you have to constantly be improving, like constantly be actively learning. He talked about just how he is kind of obsessed with reading journals. I found it very inspiring. He is so dedicated to improving himself, and he so thoroughly enjoys what he does. I think that's how you get to be a doctor of his caliber.

In addition to their teaching, attending physicians also serve—consciously or unconsciously—as role models for their learners. In the following chapter, we look at some of the ways in which our 12 attendings fulfill that responsibility. Topics include the uncertainty principle and the hidden curriculum, patience and perseverance, and mortality and joy.

MAIN POINTS

1. Attendings viewed the use of "why" questions as teaching opportunities.

2. Questions served multiple purposes including guiding learners through their thinking processes, building on knowledge through the use of hypothetical questions, and using the Socratic method to foster critical thinking.

3.   Instilling the ability to think critically about one's own decision-making process was the attendings' ultimate goal for their learners.

Further Reading

Tofade, T., Elsner, J., & Haines, S. T. (2013). Best practice strategies for effective use of questions as a teaching tool. *American Journal of Pharmaceutical Education, 77*(7), 155.

Although the use of questions is essential in the teaching process, little is known about how to effectively use questions to teach. Thus, in this review, the authors summarize a taxonomy of questions and provide strategies for formulating effective questions. Questions should be seen as teaching tools that can guide students to deeper insights and promote critical thinking.

Long, M., Blankenburg, R., & Butani, L. (2015). Questioning as a teaching tool. *Pediatrics, 135*(3), 406–408.

The authors provide an approach to questioning that aims to match questions to the learner's ability while maintaining a supportive learning environment. Using the Dreyfus and Bloom frameworks, educators can formulate questions that are learner-centric while at the same time challenging learners to think critically. Questions are a valuable teaching, learning, and assessment tool.

Brancati, F. L. (1989). The art of pimping. *Journal of the American Medical Association, 262*(1), 89–90.

In this now classic commentary, Dr. Brancati from Johns Hopkins University presents an overview of the origins and motivation of the art of pimping in the medical field. Pimping is the method of questioning in which the attending asks a series of difficult questions of the learner. The author goes on to provide a brief guide to the art of pimping by clearly defining the five key categories a pimping question may fall under: (1) arcane points of history, (2) teleology and metaphysics, (3) exceedingly broad questions, (4) eponyms, and (5) technical points of laboratory research. The author concludes that, if done correctly, the use of pimping can result in a prepared and knowledgeable learner.

Role Models

■□■

Being a role model is the most powerful form of educating.

—JOHN WOODEN

TO ONE EXTENT or another, for better or worse, attending physicians become their learners' role models. One survey found that 90% of a medical school's graduating class listed one or more physician role models.[1] The 12 outstanding attendings we interviewed and observed take this informal aspect of their teaching very seriously. They understand that their behavior, as physicians, as instructors, as human beings, will most likely be internalized and emulated by some of their learners. As a result, they continually monitor themselves, striving to make sure that they are living up to their personal and professional standards.

"I'm a big believer in role modeling," one attending told us. For her, the most important example she sets is the evident pleasure she takes in caring for patients. "There is a lot of joy-sucking that can happen in a hospital where people just get really entrenched on their gerbil wheels churning out patients," she said. "It sounds trite, but I think you should just stop and smell the roses, and I try to make sure we pay attention to that."

The former learner of another attending explained how she had inspired him to go into hospital medicine. "I learned from her how to navigate people and systems in an inpatient environment, how to work well with lots of different people. She was my role model."

In the previous chapters, we discussed the 12 attendings' creation of supportive and team-based environments and their teaching techniques. In this chapter, our focus is on some of the personal qualities the attendings model and some of the special challenges they confront in that endeavor. The ultimate goal in their role-modeling mission will be the focus of the following chapter: their treatment of patients.

Our attendings have high expectations for their team members—and for themselves. "I'm a perfectionist, and I have high standards for myself," one of the attendings said, "but I think it's really important to take each student as an individual and help them be the best they can be, not necessarily to my standards."

Even those learners who have been directly criticized by an attending and told that they are not working as hard as they could know "deep inside," a former learner said, that the attending will protect them and work to "pull their good things [out of them]."

But the 12 attendings don't cut themselves much slack as role models. "You know, he's working harder than anybody on the team," an attending's former learner said, "and that really sets the bar for how you expect yourself to work."

Here's how another former learner described his attending's approach:

He was as nice and calm as you could be with the students, the residents, and the patients, but in the background he was doing as much hard work as anybody else, checking up on the patients, checking up on us, checking up on medications, reconciliations. While all that was happening, he had a very carefree approach during rounds, like, this is easy, let's have fun. But in the background, that was never really the case. The informality makes everyone like him, makes everyone learn from him very well, and meanwhile he's very hands-on, doing things.

As teachers and physicians working in the frenetic hospital environment, our attendings must cope with frequent periods of stress and frustration, yet as role models they must strive to keep their cool. Their learners say they do so. One learner recalled a time when his attending was unhappy with the update his team provided about one of their patients; the attending ended up in the hospital at 10 P.M. "He was concerned," the learner said, "but I have never seen him get angry. Never at all."

Two learners were discussing an attending. "I did not get the sense that he lost his temper by accident," said the first. "I think he used it as a tool to indicate that what was happening was not O.K." The second learner replied: "Yeah, I've seen that, like when he says some particular thing has made him 'cranky.' He uses 'cranky' to add emphasis, right? But I haven't seen him . . . raise his voice."

One attending did admit to almost losing it when a social worker, talking with a patient, started questioning the attending's medical decisions. "I was in the team room later when I called this individual," the attending told us. "I was very much aware that the team was listening. I was clearly upset, but I wasn't unprofessional. I was kind of proud of myself."

To maintain their twofold task as physician and teacher, the 12 attendings must be models of self-discipline. That can make for a long day. "My attending gets up at 4 o'clock every morning and reads the journals," a current learner told us in admiration and wonder. His colleague added: "When I think about him, discipline comes to mind."

A key element of the attendings' self-discipline is their routine monitoring of their own performance. They understand that keeping tabs on themselves can help them achieve their goal of continuous improvement.

Our attendings make it clear to their teams that physicians can never rest on their laurels. "He is the most knowledgeable person," a learner said of his attending, "yet even he himself admits you're never perfect and you've just got to keep on learning." The attendings are constantly looking for ways to improve their skills, and their learners know it. One of the attendings told us about reviewing the literature to find articles that will "make me a better doctor and maybe a better teacher." Another spoke of his effort to live up to his own role models: "What inspired me was I had role models in my life that just 'I want to be like that' and I'm still trying to 'be like that.'"

An attending echoed the need to learn from others:

> My teaching now is better than it was five years ago, and I bet it will be better five years from now. You know, when I do something good but someone does it even better, I love to hear about it. Because, you know, you are on a personal quest to do better and better, but your own creativity is limited, and someone else's creativity is limitless.

Another attending was talking about how to improve teaching competence. His team, he said, "should go watch other attendings teach and then reflect carefully about what they learned and how it could be used to improve their own teaching skills." In fact, he went on, that's what he and the other attendings have been doing: "All of us have gotten better, I think, over the years I've been here, and in part it's because we are watching each other."

Behind the attendings' commitment to self-improvement is their core belief in the value of the larger medical enterprise. They care about their legacy as part of that enterprise. "My job is to tell you what I know and to make sure that, at the end, you know more than I do," one of the 12 attendings told us, "and to make sure that I have inspired you to do that to the people who come after you."

That is how they present themselves to their teams. "You see his devotion to a cause he feels is his calling in life," a learner said of his attending, "and you can see yourself trying your best to emulate that."

As teachers and role models, attendings need to be conscious of a force that can often work against their efforts—what one article describes as "the informal and hidden curricula that are ubiquitous in hospitals and medical schools."[2] The hidden curriculum consists of a set of values and behaviors that are seldom acknowledged but are widely accepted and practiced within a hospital, for good or for ill. It represents, in effect, another kind of role model for learners—a model that can undermine the efforts of responsible attending physicians.

In their treatment of patients, for example, the hospital's mores may emphasize efficiency over empathy, so that physicians typically pay little attention to patients' emotional concerns. Nurses may be treated as inferiors, not partners. Learners may be expected to kowtow to their attendings.

During our interviews of the 12 attendings' team members and former learners, we often encountered veiled references to the hidden curriculum. They spoke of physicians who had demeaned them in front of other people or were "so intimidating you're afraid to talk or communicate with them." They expressed relief that their attending "doesn't have this need to have the last say because of his position" or was "not about making us look bad or feel bad."

There have been a number of professional initiatives in recent years to combat a common element of the hidden curriculum, the tendency to overuse medical investigation, including diagnostic tests. The initiatives call for an end to wasteful spending, which costs an estimated $210 billion a year.[3]

As we made rounds with our attendings, we saw them modeling an attitude of less is more, prioritizing the patient's comfort and safety over extra testing. "Any labs?" one attending asked an intern. "We stopped the labs," was the response. "Oh, good," the attending commented. "Only do things that will bring value." Another attending addressed his team: "To what end are we going to put this guy through that? We could increase his delirium, and I'm not certain we could find any cancer. I'm not in favor of putting him through this procedure."

The hidden curriculum can and should be a positive factor that reinforces the values of attending physicians, but they need to be aware of the negative influence it can sometimes have on their learners and on their own behavior.

Our attendings are out front with their learners about some home truths. They never stop reminding their teams, for example, that uncertainty is an integral part of the practice of medicine. The results of a physical exam are often ambiguous, as are the results of tests and consults with experts. Not only do experienced physicians sometimes disagree about a given diagnosis, but any one of the physicians may also have a different view of the matter on any given day. Imaging and other tests can deliver ambivalent results, accompanied by incomplete computer interpretations (Figure 7.1).

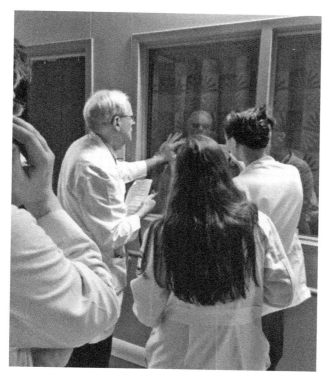

FIGURE 7.1 Attending and team looking at an electrocardiogram (ECG) during rounds.

As role models, how do the 12 attendings cope with the uncertainty factor? One of them described a patient who presented with both a bleeding lesion from metastatic cancer in the head and a big pulmonary embolism experienced a month earlier. There was no clear path forward. We asked the attending how she helped her team cope with such a situation.

"You talk about the risks and benefits on both sides of the equation," she said, "and try to then be as transparent about the decision-making process as you can. We put our heads together to come up with the best plan for the patient while recognizing that this is the risk we're about to take."

By bringing the learners into the discussion and sharing her own thought process, the attending models the collegial behavior that is most effective in resolving complex clinical problems.

We frequently heard the 12 attendings acknowledging the uncertainties of medical practice. "It's a little bit of a mystery, guys," said one. Another admitted, "Sometimes you go down a road that leads you nowhere."

A current learner told us how his attending personalizes that unpredictability. "You know the typical stories they tell: Nobody was able to figure it out, but then I came in and figured it out and everything was good. Well, the stories my attending tells are mostly about the cases where he got the thing wrong. He wants to share his mistakes with you so you can learn from them." The attending was also modeling an attitude: Mistakes are part and parcel of a profession that must cope with ambivalence; they are to be lamented, but there is no shame in sharing them for the good of the profession.

Where there is ambivalence, there is risk; where there is risk, there can be dire consequences. That's when attending physicians face some of their toughest role model challenges, when a patient they and their team have been caring for has a bad result. They have to model the appropriate behavior not just with their teams but with the patient and with the patient's family as well.

Bad outcomes can take a heavy emotional toll on individual learners and on the whole team. "I can get very emotionally invested in my patients and their families," a current learner told us, "and I know I'm going to have patients who are going to succumb to their disease. My attending really models how to deal with that so I can in the future maybe avoid physician burnout or fatigue or lack of empathy."

We observed another attending setting an example for his team on how to cope with the recent death of one of their patients:

> ATTENDING: When we have a bad outcome, we tend to go over and over it. I spend a lot of porch time thinking about it. We should reflect on what happened but not lose our confidence. The day after he died, I sat in my truck and did a personal pep talk. You have to come in and take care of the next patient and do the best you can.
>
> MEDICAL STUDENT: Do you ever go to a patient's funeral?
>
> ATTENDING: Yes, but not for me. I go if I think it will help the family or they ask me to go. You know, if it feels like your soul has been ripped out after a bad outcome, then you've done something right. You've made that connection with the patient. My job is to build communication between all of us so we feel vested in each other and our patients.

As we mentioned in Chapter 4, gallows humor, what one of our attendings called "dark humor," is a traditional coping mechanism in hospitals. Attendings and their team members make these morbid jokes to provide some relief from their day-long encounters with disease and death. We heard few of them during our observations of the 12 attendings, who are aware that gallows humor is not for everyone—and definitely not for patients. The attendings monitored their listeners' responses to all of their jokes, sensitive to any negative reactions. As a former learner noted, describing physicians with a good bedside manner, "They know how to back pedal when they sense their humor is not working." Lesson learned.

Most of the joking our attendings model is modest, situational humor. For example, we saw one of the attendings ask a patient to stick out his tongue. After the patient did so, the attending said: "You did that with such vigor, I think you're trying to tell us something."

The attendings use humor and laughter as teaching tools, as a way to keep their teams alert and involved in the learning process. But the humor is also a natural expression of something very basic about the 12 attendings, something they clearly model for their team. Here's how a former learner describes it:

> He likes being a doctor, and you can see it when he practices. He's happy doing what he is doing. It inspires us that, yes, we will be happy just by trying to help other people by being a doctor.

In the following chapter, we describe the behavior of our attendings with their patients, the most important way in which they serve their teams as role models. We will discuss, for example, their techniques for winning over patients, from using warm stethoscopes to meeting patients' emotional needs.

"He was always very gentle with patients," a former learner said of one of the 12 attendings, "and he took the time to explain things. And I think that really helped shape who I am, because that's something, if you don't see it, you don't necessarily know that it matters. And I got to see it."

MAIN POINTS

1. Attendings generally hold themselves to a higher standard than they do their learners.

2. Role modeling is an important part of the teaching process and includes demonstrating how to be a lifelong learner, maintaining professionalism in the face of adversity, and acknowledging the emotional toll caring for patients can have on oneself.

3. Humor with both learners and patients was common among the attendings, as was expressing the joys of being a doctor.

Further Reading

Branch, Jr. W. T., Kern, D., Haidet, P., Weissmann, P., Gracey, C. F., Mitchell, G., & Inui, T. (2001). Teaching the human dimensions of care in clinical settings. *Journal of the American Medical Association, 286*(9), 1067–1074.

In this article, the authors describe a climate of learning that may be lacking in the teaching of humanism. They identify

several strategies to overcome barriers to teaching humanism that include taking advantage of seminal events, such as
demonstrating how to deliver bad news; role modeling by acting; commenting on and explaining what you have done; and
using active learning skills by involving learners in tasks that
require them to use humanistic skills. However, the authors
point out that in order to implement these strategies, institutes
must first establish a climate of humanism.

Morden, N. E., Colla, C. H., Sequist, T. D., & Rosenthal, M. B.
(2014). Choosing wisely—The politics and economics of label-
ing low-value services. *New England Journal of Medicine*,
370(7), 589–592.

In this perspective, Morden and colleagues summarize
the progress made through the American Board of Internal
Medicine Foundation's "stewards of finite health care
resources" initiative. Professional organizations volunteered
to be guided through "Top Five" lists that focused on achiev-
ing practice change through improving patient health, reducing risk, and reducing costs. The effort was expanded and
launched as the Choosing Wisely campaign and demonstrates
physicians' willingness to change their role in the habitual
overuse of healthcare resources.

Saint, S., Fowler, K. E., Krein, S. L., Flanders, S. A., Bodnar, T.
W., Young, E., & Moseley, R. H. (2013). An academic hospitalist model to improve healthcare worker communication
and learner education: Results from a quasi-experimental
study at a Veterans Affairs Medical Center. *Journal of Hospital
Medicine*, *8*(12), 702–710.

In this multimodal systems redesign of one of four medical teams in a Midwestern Veterans Affairs center, the authors
tested various approaches to improving healthcare worker
communication and learner education. The authors found
that the intervention team's attendings received higher teaching scores and that third-year medical students scored significantly higher on their shelf exam, indicating that a focus
on improving communication and enhancing learner education is possible without increasing patient length of stay or
readmission rates.

8

The Sacred Act of Healing

■□■

The greatest mistake in the treatment of diseases is that there are physicians for the body and physicians for the soul, although the two cannot be separated.

—PLATO

IN RECENT YEARS, patient-centered care has become a key goal of the American medical establishment. The Institute of Medicine, for example, in its 2001 report, "Crossing the Quality Chasm," issued a call for doctors to be "respectful of and responsive to individual patient preferences, needs, and values" and to ensure that "patient values guide all clinical decisions."[1] In other words, the physician-centered model of hospital care must yield to one in which the patient's experience of illness is now of equal concern, at least, with that of the doctor's. Powerful support for the patient-centered movement has come from the widespread redefinition of the patient as a consumer whose satisfaction has become a marketplace necessity.

Such concern for the centrality of the patient has been heard before. Back in the 1920s, for example, when Francis W. Peabody, an eminent physician, was writing his influential essays and books, he addressed the common complaint that the era's medical school graduates were more engaged with the mechanisms of disease than with the care of their patients. He wrote:

The good physician knows his patients through and through, and his knowledge is bought dearly. Time, sympathy, and understanding must be lavishly dispensed, but the reward is to be found in that personal bond which forms the greatest satisfaction of the practice of medicine.[2]

That same dedication is a core characteristic of our 12 attending physicians. It is reflected in a comment of one of the attendings, a comment that might well serve as a message to medical students everywhere. "The patient's room is a sacred place," he said, "and it's a privilege for us to be in there. And if we don't earn that privilege, then we don't get to go there."

This chapter shows how our attendings care for their patients in that sacred place—and serve as role models for their learners in the process. The attendings' behavior with their patients often establishes the standard that learners will follow throughout their professional careers.

Each encounter we witnessed between one of our attendings and a patient was, of course, a unique occasion, but many of them were markedly similar to the session set forth here. The attending was a skillful examiner and interviewer, weighing the patient's symptoms and history and then deciding on a course of action. With his empathy and sense of humor, he established a positive connection with both mother and patient that eased the way for the examination and led to new information about the patient's family history.

We entered the patient's room, and the attending quickly struck up a conversation with the patient's mother. They spoke about how many children she had and laughingly discussed whether the patient was a good son or not. The attending showed us the patient's fingernails, which were hyperpigmented. "You should see how bad my toe-nails are," the patient said. When the attending wanted to check his feet, the patient resisted. "My own wife hasn't seen my toes for 10 years," he said, but he eventually relented.

ATTENDING: Those aren't so bad. Do you work some-where where your feet get wet?

PATIENT: I'm a cook.

ATTENDING: So water is probably splashing on your feet. That's what happens. Are you lifting things at work?

PATIENT: I can't do that anymore.

[Additional discussion about work activities performed.]

ATTENDING [To PATIENT]: I was thinking about you last night, and I want the GI [gastrointestinal] people to see you.

The patient's mother asked the attending whether her son had cancer, pointing out that it had struck both sides of his family. Her son had been extensively evaluated without showing any signs of cancer, the attending replied, but he repeated his call for a GI consultation.

As we all started to leave the room, we heard the attend-ing say to the patient's mother, "I know you are worried about your boy, but we're taking care of him."

By this time, everyone else was out the door, but the attending stayed to have a few private words with the patient's mother.

In matters large and small, the 12 attendings are aware that they are role models for their learners, and they behave accordingly. Before and after every patient, for example, they used antiseptic gel or washed their hands with soap and water, depending on the circumstances. They wore gloves when examining patients' wounds. They kept their stethoscopes clean.

The attendings were careful in every aspect of their clinical work. When a team dove right into the rhythm of a newly arrived electrocardiogram (EKG), their attending called a halt: "First, make sure it's for this patient. There's nothing worse than going through a whole EKG to find out it wasn't your patient."

Our attendings were also thorough, especially when examining patients. They warmed their stethoscopes before use and auscultated directly on the patient's body. "She does it the right way every time," a current learner said of his attending. "You can see other attendings auscultate over gowns or clothing, but you see she's doing it the way it was taught and that's what you want to emulate."

During the physical exam, the attendings each had his or her individual techniques. "He has a very distinct way," a former learner said of his attending, "deciding which parts are the most important to do to go down the diagnostic algorithm of why this patient has shoulder pain."

But all of the attendings placed great emphasis on the importance of the physical exam, and they were persistent questioners on the trail of a diagnosis and a cause:

ATTENDING: Do you have any trouble breathing?

PATIENT: No.

ATTENDING: Do you ever feel short of breath?

PATIENT: No.

ATTENDING: Have you ever smoked?

PATIENT: No.

ATTENDING: How about anyone in the house?

PATIENT: No.

ATTENDING: Growing up?

PATIENT: Oh, yeah. Everyone in my family smoked but me.

In developing diagnoses, the attendings urged their learners to "prioritize," to look for the most probable answers or, as a current learner put it, "the big things you hang your hat on as your first pass." At the same time, our attendings demonstrated a keen ability to develop differential diagnoses beyond those big things.

"She finds relevant details that other people wouldn't think important," a current learner said of his attending. "If you presume that certain relationships can exist, you'll see them when they do. And if you limit yourself to things that are very scripted, you're only going to see those things. She's good at doing the former; she doesn't do the latter."

As discussed in earlier chapters, the 12 attendings are not shy about admitting what they don't know. When they lack a clear diagnosis or are stumped as to the appropriate treatment, they will call for an expert consultation. But automatic consultation is not their default position.

A former learner described his attending: "He takes ownership and responsibility. He is really, 'I know what's going on and I'll consult you when I *really* need you, not just for the sake of it.'"

The attendings want to get their patients up from bed and walking as soon as possible. "It's better than laboratory tests, fancy CT [computed tomography] scans," a former learner said, echoing his attending. "Walking the patient around the room, pushing the pole, closing the back of the gown so they don't expose themselves to everybody, and making sure the Foley is not pulling anything. It's not always an easy thing to do, but my attending would do it all the time."

The 12 attendings' focus on the patient's physical condition doesn't end with a firm diagnosis and a stable patient. They are constantly looking for new ways to think through the patient's situation, taking nothing for granted—in a sense, looking for trouble. One of the attendings asked his team where their diabetic patient was giving himself his insulin shot. Too many times in the same spot, he warned, and there would be a danger of neuropathy and of shortening the medicine's half-life.

"I actually used to like going in cold in the morning with no clue about what's coming," one of our attendings told us. Now, like most of the other 11, he reads up on new patients before he meets with his team. Knowing patients' lab values and medical history saves time on rounds, and time is of the essence given the hectic pace required of house staff in today's hospitals. It means that the up-to-date attendings can, in the words of a current learner, "quickly identify subtle differences in the way patients present and be aware of some of their laboratory abnormalities that may potentially be related to their chief complaint." And it helps attendings plan their mornings more efficiently because they know which patients have more complex problems and will thus require extra time.

The attendings also bone up on their patients because of duty hour restrictions. "You have to have a full picture of what's going on with a patient before most of the team who know the patient go home at 11 A.M.," one of the attendings explained. "It's impossible for the single team member left with knowledge of the patients to handle all the questions and calls."

The fact that their attendings are so knowledgeable about their patients can be a spur to learners. "Maybe other attendings might be a little more lax with what happened 10 years ago and wouldn't push us to look as deeply into charts," a current learner said. "Our attending always knows what's going on in-depth, and that pushes all of us to do the same."

Patient-centered care can yield significant benefits for both physicians and patients. When traditionally passive patients become active participants in their care, good things can happen. For our attendings, the good things happen at the bedside. "Doing it outside of the room, going through lab values in front of a computer, you lose the connection with the patient," a current learner said, reflecting his attending's views. "This is a person we are treating. These are her lab values, and this is her life right now. It's everything to her. She should be part of the discussion."

When physician and patient talk, the physician explains the patient's condition and treatment plan. The informed patient shares old and new details about her condition and her personal history, aiding the management of her case during her hospital stay and thereafter. The closer connection makes it possible for the physician to convince the patient to take her appropriate medications and curtail counterproductive behavior. It can also convince her to give the attending useful feedback about her treatment in general and about the behavior of the resident team.

The 12 attendings create this kind of relationship by demonstrating, in dozens of ways, their empathy and respect for every patient. They smile as they enter a patient's room, seeking to set a positive and friendly tone for the encounter.

They introduce themselves and their team to the patient if it's a first visit. They quickly size up the situation of the patient, looking to her comfort. "Is the sunlight bothering your eyes?" one of the attendings asked a patient and proceeded to close the blinds. They will usually find a way to create a pleasant verbal exchange with the patient, tailoring their approach to the individual.

"All right, rock star," an attending said to a patient. "Tell me the story behind all those bracelets you're wearing." Laughing, the patient showed the attending his favorite. The attending read it aloud, "Don't be stupid," and added, "Words we can all live by."

One of our attendings has traveled widely in the U.S. and he often starts conversations with patients by asking where they come from because, chances are, he's been there and can share his impressions. He's also been in the military, so his opening gambit with veterans is, "What branch of the service were you in?" With younger patients, the attendings may ask the name of their pet. With elderly patients, they are more likely to ask them, "What was the most memorable moment in your life?" An attending told us, "I just show patients I'm interested in them as people, and you can see the effect it has. It's part of being a good doctor."

To put patients at ease, our attendings will often use humor. They make fun of themselves or of team members. "This guy," an attending said, turning to his patient, "was sick when he came in. He was soft and weak, like one of our interns." Otherwise, their humor tends to be gentle, especially when it directly involves patients. When a patient said, "I thought you weren't coming," an attending replied, "We had to see the sick people first."

The attendings' humor is typically spontaneous and situational. An attending, struggling with a bed rail and a mattress that was moving up and down, complained, "Jeez, this bed is like a Venus flytrap." A former learner recalled rounding all through the football playoffs: "With every patient, even the Spanish-speaking ones, the attending would be like, 'Hey, can we change this channel? The Texans are playing, you know, American football!' And we would change the channel, and the patients would start laughing."

During the physical examination, the attendings seek to make sure the process is as free from discomfort and embarrassment as possible. Their exam technique is thorough but gentle and informative. We listened in on one of our attendings at the bedside: "A few of us are going to listen to you this morning. I'm going on the other side so you'll have one of us on each side of you.... Can you turn your head? We want to look at your neck.... This is like a gas gauge and will let us know if you are full or empty of fluid." Curtains are drawn around the bed for privacy and gowns are closed back up when the exam is over. The attendings will often use a comforting touch, particularly at the end of the exam.

Their empathy becomes most evident, though, when the patient is in severe pain. In one instance, an attending stayed by the patient's side, stroking her arm, telling her to breathe slowly, while sending for more pain medication. "I'm sorry you're in so much pain," the attending said several times. When leaving, the attending asked an intern to stay with the patient until the new medication was administered.

The final stage of a team's departure receives careful attention from the 12 attendings. As one of them said, "You make sure the room is how you left it when you walked in. You turn off the lights if they were off; you take care of the bedrails; you fix the TV volume." They also offer patients a pleasant, upbeat farewell along the lines of "A pleasure meeting you" and, yes, "Have a nice day."

As part of their dedication to patient-centeredness, our attendings keep their patients in the loop. After the physical exam, for instance, the attendings would tell a patient that they were going to "talk shop" with their team to discuss their findings, but would translate what was said into layman's language after the shop talk. To make sure their patients understood their diagnosis and treatment plan, the attendings would regularly ask patients, "Tell me what we're up to," or "Tell me what our plan is."

In the following exchange, one of our attendings explained to a patient and his wife the procedure being considered to prevent blood clots from going from his legs to his lungs.

ATTENDING: Do you play badminton?

WIFE: I have.

ATTENDING: So have I, and I bet I could beat you [he says jokingly]. But you know the little birdie? Well, this procedure we're thinking about, there's a net that looks like the birdie and it would be inside him and it's used to catch all the blood clots. Doing that would keep a situation like this [pulmonary embolism] from happening again, and he would feel better. He does have to be on Coumadin the rest of his life so no more Mixed Martial Arts fighting or throwing plates at his head. If you get mad at him, you can kick him below the knee.

[Conversation continued with the attending asking about another family member who was also diagnosed with the same clotting disorder. The attending recommended they discuss it with their children's pediatrician since the disorder could be hereditary.]

In addition to demonstrating the attending's desire to keep his patients informed, the preceding exchange illustrates other elements of his patient-centered approach including his use of humor and his concern for the patient's family. In fact, the 12 attendings are fully committed to keeping their patients' families up to date on patients' condition and prognosis. "He's always having a family meeting or calling a patient's wife to tell her what we did today and the plan," a former learner recalled of his attending.

Our attendings are also in touch with their patients' outpatient physicians, alerting them to their patients' presence in the hospital and keeping them aware of major developments.

When they talk with their patients, the attendings often kneel down or sit on a stool in order to talk eye to eye (Figure 8.1). "I feel you're able to connect with people much better that way than if you're towering over them," one of the attendings said. She went on: "It's a horrible power dynamic to be sick and someone's standing over you telling you things."

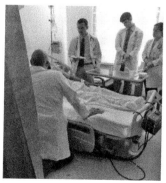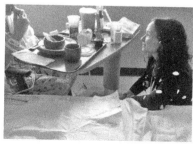

FIGURE 8.1 Attendings kneeling at patient's bedside.

Another attending told us that kneeling by the bedside sent patients a message: "You think it's uncomfortable? Damn right! It hurts." The point of the message? "It's just to remind them, we don't lord over the patient," he said. "This is their place."

During their talks with patients, the attendings spoke calmly and slowly. And they listened, patiently and carefully. A former learner described his attending "sitting through everything the patients said, even when they were saying a million things that didn't really make a whole lot of sense."

Physicians can learn a great deal from listening to their patients. They learn about aspects of the patients' medical history and their family's medical history that can shed fresh light on current medical conditions and treatments. Physicians can also get a line on patients' personalities, which can help physicians deal with recalcitrant patients. Here's how one of our attendings applied that knowledge in coping with a patient who had just undergone open heart surgery but refused to take pain medications: "Someone took a saw to your breastbone. You're not a wuss if you need pain meds. And it will make it a lot easier for you to do your rehabilitation." The patient agreed to try some pain meds.

Knowledge of the details of patients' lives can also be invaluable in planning for their departure and outpatient existence. "We have a patient who is very sick," a current learner told us, "and our attending learned that the patient's wife was admitted at another institution in the same city. Right away, he realized that was going to be a problem when the patient went home. Who would take care of him? So we had our social worker and case manager talk with [the other institution's social worker] to work out a solution."

Our attendings start thinking about their patients' hospital discharge as soon as they are admitted to the hospital. A current learner described her attending's early outpatient focus: "It seems like she always has a plan, like, 'Oh, by the way, when this patient leaves, they're going to need this, this, and this. You should start on that now.'"

The attendings' outpatient concern extended beyond medical care to encompass the financial needs of their patients. We heard an attending talking to her team: "What was the purpose of our palliative care conversation yesterday? To consider the patient's insurance. She has Medicaid that might affect the amount of palliative care [she is eligible for]. . . ."

During our interviews, we talked with a current learner about his attending as role model and the special relationship his attending creates with his patients. "My experience is that patients don't really know whether they're being treated appropriately," the learner said. "They don't know that this medication is better than that medication for such and such a reason. My attending actually is just the best at managing patients medically. But he has also gone beyond the traditional scope of a physician in the sense that he is meeting patients' emotional needs—and that's pretty rare. It's something I'm really hoping to take with me."

Up to this point in the book, we have reported our observations of the 12 outstanding attending physicians, trusting that our readers would want to follow in the attendings' eminent footsteps. In the next and final chapter, we have taken a different tack. We have recast our most important findings as recommendations. We hope that readers will find this more direct and simplified form of value in the evolution of their own careers as attendings.

MAIN POINTS

1. Attendings treated their patients with respect, empathy, and understanding. Even though their encounters might be brief, attendings made it a priority to get to know their patients and build rapport. Developing these relationships helped the team plan for the patient's care both within and outside the hospital.

2. Attendings spent time explaining to patients, in layman's language, what they were thinking and how they were approaching the patient's treatment. They often sat down or kneeled when speaking to patients so they could be on the same level.

3. In order to stave off readmissions, attendings looked beyond the issues that brought patients into the hospital in the first place for problems that could be addressed while the patient was still hospitalized.

Further Reading

Mullan, F. (2001). A founder of quality assessment encounters a troubled system firsthand. *Health Affairs*, *20*(1), 137–141.

In this article, Avedis Donabedian, a physician, scholar, and poet, is interviewed by Fitzhugh Mullan shortly before his death. The topics covered included Donabedian's reflections on being a patient, his personal feeling on the quality of care he had received, and his sense of confidence in the day-to-day management of his care. In response to a question regarding his feelings about the rapid commercialization of healthcare in recent years, Donabedian responded, "Ultimately, the secret quality is love. You have to love your patient, you have to love your profession, you have to love your God. If you have love, you can then work backward to monitor and improve the system."

Peabody, F. W. (1927). The care of the patient. *Journal of the American Medical Association, 88*(12), 877–882.

In this essay, Peabody stresses that one cannot simply become a skillful practitioner of medicine in the time allotted for training in medical school. He emphasizes that medicine is not a trade to be learned but rather a profession to be entered; it is a profession that requires continuous study and prolonged experience taking care of patients. Peabody addresses three main topics: the importance of individualizing medical care, a call for awareness that hospitalization can be a dehumanizing experience, and the care of patients whose cause of symptoms cannot be diagnosed.

Hartzband, P., & Groopman, J. (2009). Keeping the patient in the equation—Humanism and health care reform. *New England Journal of Medicine, 361*(6), 554–555.

In this article, the authors discuss two movements that have emerged in recent years: medical humanism and evidence-based practice. Although both movements aim to improve patient care, their approaches to accomplishing this goal differ. Humanism aims to understand the patient as a person, focusing on individual values, goals, and preferences, whereas evidence-based practice aims to put medicine on a firmer scientific footing using data and clinical guidance to standardize procedures and therapies. They point out the obstacles these two movements may face, as well as how they may coalesce rather than conflict with one another.

Putting It All Together

■□■

*He who studies medicine without books sails an
uncharted sea, but he who studies medicine without
patients does not go to sea at all.*

—WILLIAM OSLER

ATTENDING PHYSICIANS HAVE always borne a weighty
responsibility. To a large extent, they are accountable for the
quality of their learners' clinical skills and knowledge and,
thus, for the level of medical care received by each succeed-
ing generation of patients. But today, they confront unprecedented challenges.

They have less time to spend with their teams because
of new limits on learners' work hours. Because patients' hospital stays are shorter, attendings' and learners' time with
individual patients has shrunk even as the patient population has grown substantially sicker. Meanwhile, attendings
must adjust to the hospitals' seismic shift from a physician-
centered to a patient-centered mindset.

Our study of 12 outstanding attending physicians was
intended to help today's attendings manage these new and
daunting circumstances. We believed that a detailed, mul-
tiperspective description of the instructional and clinical
methods of these remarkable attendings would yield a trove

of practical, actionable advice for internal medicine physicians and physicians-in-training.

In this final chapter, we have recapped that advice, encompassing many of the 12 attendings' most important strategies and practices.

CREATE A SUPPORTIVE TEAM ENVIRONMENT

As an attending physician, you need to set high standards for your team and make sure that team members live up to them. But the performance anxiety that so often accompanies educational standards is not conducive to rational thinking and the learning process. In your presence, you want your team to feel safe and comfortable, during table rounds and—especially—patient rounds. In your absence, you want your team to feel safe and comfortable enough to call you if there is concern for the patient. To maximize learning, you want the team atmosphere to be cooperative and trusting rather than competitive. Here are some of the ways to achieve those ends.

Develop Personal Relationships

Get to know your team members by asking about their life experiences and being open about your own. Address them by their first names. Use humor to lighten the atmosphere and make rounds more informal and enjoyable; self-deprecating humor is most effective. If team members are comfortable with you personally, they will feel safe and comfortable on rounds.

Keep Interactions Positive

Listen carefully to learners' input and respond thoughtfully (Figure 9.1). Feedback is necessary, but try to keep it from being embarrassing to the learners; as a general rule, major criticisms should be delivered in private. When team members are presenting, let them talk without interruption. Their mistakes should be viewed by learners as an essential element of their education. You can encourage that view by using your own past mistakes to illustrate your teaching—and to demonstrate to learners that clinical medicine is inherently subject to uncertainty and error.

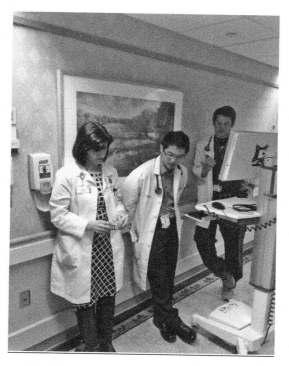

FIGURE 9.1 Attending listening intently to learner's presentation.

Tailor Your Teaching

The members of your team vary in terms of their experience and their learning level. You need to recognize these differences and adapt your instruction accordingly. Don't ask team members questions you know they cannot answer. Assign them tasks they can fulfill and learn from.

Be a Learner

Your team should understand that, as a physician and a role model, you never stop learning. Position yourself as a *member* of the team rather than the *leader* of the team (many of the attending physicians made it explicitly clear that the senior resident ran the team). Make it clear to team members that they should feel free to ask you questions and even respectfully disagree with your findings because challenges can lead to new learning. Admit when you do not know something, and share how you intend to find out about it.

DELIVER TEAM-BASED LEARNING

Put the team in charge of patient care while demonstrating to team members that you have their backs. Challenge them to question every diagnosis and every treatment plan, to develop and test multiple hypotheses and alternatives. Ideally, learners will walk away from their time spent with you understanding the value of pressure-testing presumed diagnoses and believing in the "Reagan Doctrine" as applied to patient care: Trust but verify.

Focus on Your Team's Thought Processes

Instead of lectures filled with numerous facts for them to memorize, engage members in discussions of a few key points. Instead of simply giving them answers, ask them to explain, step by step, how they arrived at a particular conclusion. Use the Socratic method of questioning to explore their understanding of the material and guide them toward the best answers.

Share Your Own Thought Processes

Tell the team your reasoning in determining the diagnosis or treatment of a patient. You want team members to learn how seasoned physicians go about that task and to build their own analytical framework.

Expand the Team

Include allied health professionals in team discussions, give them full respect, and seek their insights and direction in patients' plan of care. Nurses, in particular, can provide unique observations and perceptions of their patients. Pharmacists and social workers can make major contributions. Demonstrate the value that these professionals bring to patient care.

DELIVER PATIENT-CENTERED TEACHING

Your most important teaching takes place bedside. As your team's role model, you need to be aware that you are setting their standards for safe patient care. That means washing your hands before and after every patient visit and putting the stethoscope directly on the skin rather than over the patient's gown when listening to the lungs or heart. It requires that you put the socks back on the patient after examining his feet. It means being enthusiastic about your role as physician and teacher.

Know Your Patients

Before heading out on rounds with your team, you should have reviewed the medical records of each patient (or at least those who are the most ill). By doing so, you will know some of the key teaching points that will arise during rounds and what supporting articles you can suggest. You will also have a sense of where the team may go wrong, a prime teaching opportunity. And your foreknowledge will enable you to speed up rounds, aiding the team members' time management. Lessons learned at bedside are well remembered.

Develop Rapport with Patients

When patients like you and trust you, they are more cooperative, both in providing needed information and during physical examination. Greet them by name, relax them with jokes or chit-chat, include them and their family in discussions, explain complicated medical concepts, listen to them carefully, and sit down so you are at eye level when speaking with them. Be kind: help them change positions during examinations, be aware of their modesty, empathize with their discomfort. A touch, a smile, a bit of humility, can go a long way.

Plan for Patients' Future

When patients first arrive on the ward, start your team thinking about their departure. What kind of insurance does the patient have, and will it do the job? How will she get from hospital to home? Is there anyone at home who can take care of her? Should a team member stay in touch with her by telephone? Teach them to treat all their patients as if they were family members.

CLOSING THOUGHT

Clinical educators fulfill an important role in our healthcare system. To be a great attending means not only passing along medical knowledge but also modeling what it means to be a physician in today's healthcare environment. Thus, we leave you with a quote from one of the attendings that represents how the attendings in this study viewed their role as both doctor and teacher:

> I think [learners] have to know that you love being a teacher—
> without declaring it. It has to be obvious. They have to know
> you care about the craft—the craft of being a doctor.

Further Reading

Wiese, J. (2010). *Teaching in the Hospital*. Philadelphia, PA: ACP Press.
   In this useful book edited by one of our 12 attendings, the authors provide hospital-based educators with the tools and techniques to be successful in dispensing effective clinical education. Each chapter focuses on a different aspect of teaching and provides examples on such topics as how to establish and communicate expectations and responsibilities; how to conduct rounds in a way that ensures that education complements patient care; how to enhance learning by using illustrations, analogies, mnemonics, and other tricks of the trade; and how to coach learners in the science of clinical reasoning. Clinical problem-based teaching scripts are also provided.

Ludmerer, K. M. (2014). *Let Me Heal: The Opportunity to Preserve Excellence in American Medicine*. New York: Oxford University Press.
   The author, physician, and historian Kenneth Ludmerer provides an encompassing history of graduate medical education in the U.S. from its inception to the current day. The author demonstrates how it has changed in response to internal as well as external forces. Ludmerer calls on those within the profession to seize opportunities to improve medical education and, thus, patient care.

Irby, D. M. (1995). Teaching and learning in ambulatory care settings: A thematic review of the literature. *Academic Medicine*, *70*(10), 898–931.
   The author reviews research literature (between 1980 and 1994) on the topic of teaching and learning in ambulatory care settings. The reviewed studies suggest that education in ambulatory care clinics was limited. Case discussions were short in duration and involved little teaching, and attendings provided almost no feedback. The author recommended several strategies to facilitate learning in ambulatory care settings including increasing contact with faculty members, encouraging collaborative and self-directed learning, and strengthening assessment and feedback procedures.

APPENDIX: THE 12 ATTENDINGS

GURPREET DHALIWAL, MD

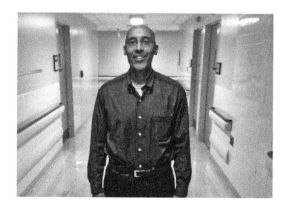

Gurpreet Dhaliwal, MD, is a clinician-educator and Professor of Medicine at the University of California at San Francisco (UCSF). He is the site director of the internal medicine clerkships at the San Francisco VA Medical Center, where he teaches medical students and residents in the emergency department, urgent care clinic, inpatient wards, outpatient clinic, and morning report. His academic interests are the cognitive processes underlying diagnostic reasoning, clinical problem-solving, and the study of diagnostic expertise. He has received numerous teaching awards including the Kaiser Award for Teaching Excellence at UCSF and the national Alpha Omega Alpha Robert J. Glaser Distinguished Teaching Award. Dr. Dhaliwal was profiled in a 2012 *New York Times* article as "one of the most skillful clinical diagnosticians in practice today."

Dr. Dhaliwal attended Northwestern University Medical School and was a resident and chief medical resident at UCSF.

JEANNE FARNAN, MD, MHPE

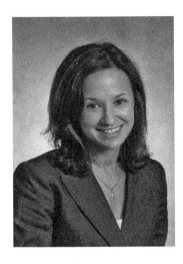

Jeanne Farnan, MD, MHPE, is Associate Professor of Medicine and Assistant Dean for Curricular Development and Evaluation at the University of Chicago Pritzker School of Medicine. Dr. Farnan is also Director of Clinical Skills Education and the Medical Director of the Clinical Performance Center. She has received the Pre-Clinical Teacher of the Year Award at the University of Chicago and has written extensively on medical professionalism and education.

Dr. Farnan received her medical degree from the University of Chicago Pritzker School of Medicine and was a resident at the University of Chicago. She received her Masters of Health Professions Education from the University of Illinois, Chicago.

SARAH HARTLEY, MD

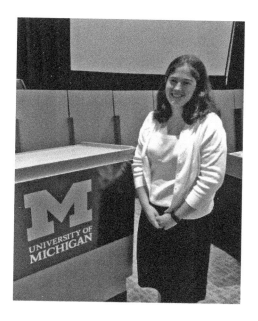

Sarah Hartley, MD, is Associate Director of the Internal Medicine Residency Program, Assistant Professor of Internal Medicine, and a hospitalist at the University of Michigan. She has received teaching awards at the University of Michigan from both medical students and residents, including the Marvin Pollard Award for Outstanding Teaching of Residents.

Dr. Hartley received her medical degree from Wayne State University School of Medicine, where she also served as a resident and chief medical resident.

ROBERT HIRSCHTICK, MD

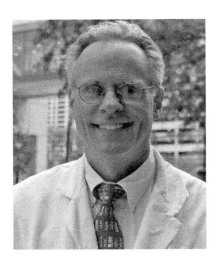

Robert Hirschtick, MD, is Associate Professor of Medicine at the Feinberg School of Medicine, Northwestern University, and the medicine clerkship site director at Chicago's Jesse Brown VA Medical Center. He has won numerous teaching awards including the Outstanding Clinical Teacher Award, the Robert J. Winter Clinical Teacher Award, the George Joost Award for Outstanding Clinical Teacher, and the "Teaching Hall of Fame" Award. He is a frequent contributor to "A Piece of My Mind" in the *Journal of the American Medical Association.*

Dr. Hirschtick received his medical degree from the University of Illinois College of Medicine and did his residency at Evanston Hospital/Northwestern.

DANIEL P. HUNT, MD

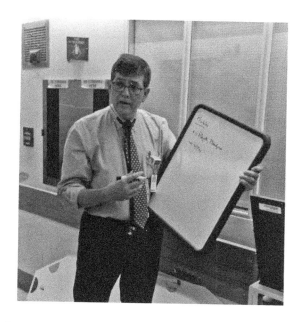

Daniel P. Hunt, MD, is Division Director of Hospital Medicine and Professor of Medicine at Emory University. He has been awarded more than 35 major teaching awards, including the Alfred Kranes Award for Excellence in Clinical Teaching from Massachusetts General Hospital, Best Clinical Instructor Award from Harvard Medical School, and the Society of Hospital Medicine's Award for Excellence in Teaching. Dr. Hunt has been the primary discussant for five "Clinicopathologic Case Conferences" published in the *New England Journal of Medicine* and has served as the unknown case discussant at national conferences.

Dr. Hunt received his medical degree from Vanderbilt University School and completed his internal medicine residency at Vanderbilt, with his third year at Baylor College of Medicine.

ROBERT MAYCOCK, MD

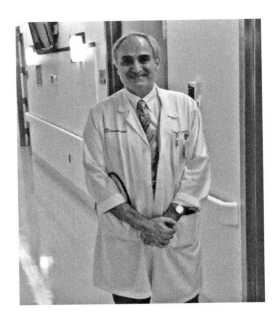

Robert Mayock, MD, is an attending physician for inpatient medicine teaching services at the Cleveland Clinic. He has won numerous teaching awards including being a five-time recipient of the Cleveland Clinic Department of Medicine Teacher of the Year Award and the Bruce Hubbard Stewart Fellowship Award for his humanistic approach to the practice of medicine.

Dr. Mayock received his medical degree from Case Western Reserve University and did his residency at the Indiana University Medical Center.

BENJAMIN MBA, MBBS, MRCP

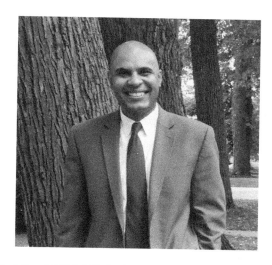

Benjamin Mba, MBBS, MRCP (UK), is Associate Chair of Medicine for Faculty Development and Associate Program Director of the Internal Medicine Residency Program at the John H. Stroger, Jr. Hospital of Cook County Chicago (former Cook County Hospital). He is also Associate Professor of Medicine at Rush University Medical Center. Dr. Mba is a three-time recipient of the Sir William Osler Award for teaching of internal medicine from the Department of Medicine at Stroger Hospital, a four-time recipient of the Division of Hospital Medicine's Cooker Award for inpatient medicine teaching and team leadership, and a two-time recipient of the Department of Medicine Medical Student Education Award.

Dr. Mba graduated from medical school in Nigeria. He initially completed an internal medicine residency training program in the United Kingdom before relocating to the U.S. He completed a second medicine residency program at the Cook County Hospital in Chicago, where he also served as a chief medical resident.

STEVEN MCGEE, MD

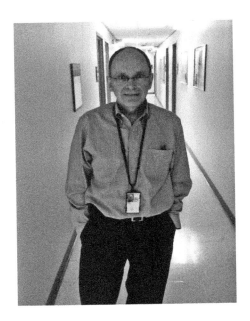

Steven McGee, MD, is Professor of Medicine at the University of Washington in Seattle and a Staff Physician at the Seattle VA Medical Center. He has won numerous teaching awards, including the Marvin Turck Outstanding Teaching Award, Teacher Superior in Perpetuity Award, the Margaret Anderson Award, two Attending-of-the-Year Awards, the Paul Beeson Teaching Award, and the National Alpha Omega Alpha Distinguished Teacher Award. He has published extensively on bedside rounding and evidence-based diagnosis, including the highly acclaimed book *Evidence-Based Physical Diagnosis*.

Dr. McGee is a graduate of Washington University School of Medicine in St. Louis, and he completed his internship, residency, chief residency, and fellowship in infectious diseases at the University of Washington School of Medicine in Seattle.

E. LEE POYTHRESS, MD

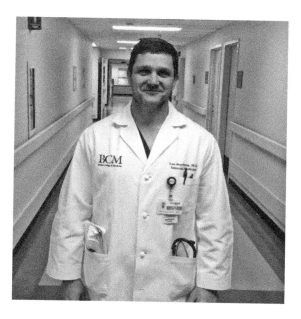

E. Lee Poythress, MD, is an Associate Professor of Medicine at Baylor College of Medicine in Houston. He has won numerous teaching awards, including being the six-time recipient of the Department of Internal Medicine Outstanding Faculty Educator Award and twice honored with the Baylor College of Medicine Medical School Outstanding Faculty Award. In 2016, he was inducted into the Baylor College of Medicine Medical School "Teaching Hall of Fame."

Dr. Poythress received his medical degree from the University of Virginia School of Medicine. He completed an internal medicine residency and geriatrics fellowship at the Baylor College of Medicine.

CHRISTINE SEIBERT, MD

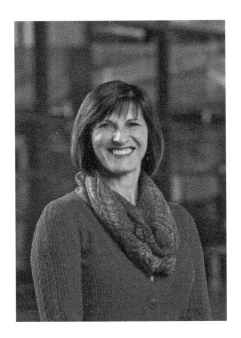

Christine Seibert, MD, is Associate Dean for Medical Student Education and Services at the University of Wisconsin School of Medicine and Public Health, as well as a Professor of Medicine. She was the recipient of the UW-Madison Chancellor's Hilldale Award for Excellence in Teaching and the School of Medicine and Public Health's Dean's Teaching Award. Dr. Seibert practices primary care general internal medicine in addition to her ward attending duties.

Dr. Seibert received her medical degree from Northwestern University. She completed an internship and residency in internal medicine at Brigham and Women's Hospital in Boston.

LAWRENCE M. TIERNEY, JR., MD

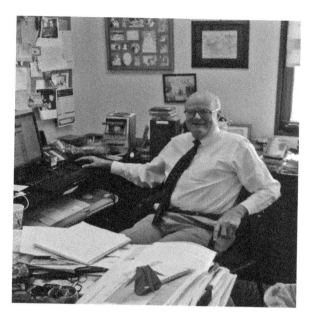

Lawrence M. Tierney, Jr., MD, serves as Professor of Medicine at the University of California at San Francisco (UCSF) School of Medicine and is the Associate Chief of Medicine at the San Francisco VA Medical Center. He has received countless teaching awards, approximately one per year for the past four decades, including the Kaiser Award and the UCSF Distinction in Teaching Award. He has been a visiting professor at more than 100 institutions around the world and is widely hailed as a master diagnostician.

Dr. Tierney—aka "LT"—received his medical degree from the University of Maryland School of Medicine. He did his residency training at both Emory and UCSF, and he completed a chief residency at UCSF.

JEFF WIESE, MD

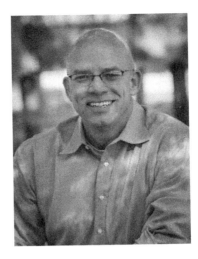

Jeff Wiese, MD, is Professor of Medicine and the Senior Associate Dean for Graduate Medical Education at the Tulane University Health Sciences Center. He is also Chief of the Charity Medical Service and the Director of the Tulane Internal Medicine Residency Program. He has won more than 50 teaching awards, including being a six-time winner of Tulane's Attending of the Year Award. His other awards include the Society of Hospital Medicine's Education Award, the Accreditation Council for Graduate Medical Education (ACGME)'s Parker Palmer Courage to Teach Award, the Association of American Medical Colleges (AAMC)'s Robert J. Glaser Distinguished Teacher Award, the American College of Physicians (ACP)'s Walter J. McDonald Award, and the Society of General Internal Medicine's Mid-Career Mentorship Award. He is the author of the book *Teaching in the Hospital*.

Dr. Wiese received his medical degree from Johns Hopkins School of Medicine and completed his internal medicine residency, chief residency, and a medical education fellowship at the University of California at San Francisco.

REFERENCES

Chapter 1: Teaching Medicine

1. FACTS: Applicants, matriculants, enrollment, graduates, M.D.-Ph.D., and residency applicants data. (2016). Retrieved from https://aamc.org/download/54360/data/whatrolesdoth-fulfill.pdf
2. Why teaching hospitals are important to all Americans. (2016). Retrieved from https://news.aamc.org/for-the-media/article/teaching-hospitals-important-americans/
3. Culliton, B. J. (2006). Extracting knowledge from science: A conversation with Elias Zerhouni. *Health Affairs, 25*(3), w94–w103.
4. Castiglioni, A., Shewchuk, R. M., Willett, L. L., Heudebert, G. R., & Centor, R. M. (2008). A pilot study using nominal group technique to assess residents' perceptions of successful attending rounds. *Journal of General Internal Medicine, 23*(7), 1060–1065.
5. Elnicki, D. M., & Cooper, A. (2005). Medical students' perceptions of the elements of effective inpatient teaching by attending physicians and housestaff. *Journal of General Internal Medicine, 20*(7), 635–639.

6. Mann, K. V. (2011). Theoretical perspectives in medical education: Past experience and future possibilities. *Medical Education*, *45*(1), 60–68.
7. Marshall, C., & Rossman, G. B. (2011). *Designing Qualitative Research*. Sage.

Chapter 2: Why Study Attending Physicians?

1. Wachter, R. M., & Goldman, L. (1996). The emerging role of "hospitalists" in the American health care system. *New England Journal of Medicine*, *335*(7), 514–517.
2. Creating the hospital of the future: The implications for hospital-focused physician practice. (2012). Retrieved from http://www.ahaphysicianforum.org/files/pdf/hospital-of-the-future.pdf.
3. Harkin, B., Webb, T. L., Chang, B. P., Prestwich, A., Conner, M., Kellar, I., Benn, Y., & Sheeran, P. (2016). Does monitoring goal progress promote goal attainment? A meta-analysis of the experimental evidence. *Psychological Bulletin*, *142*(2), 198–229.

Chapter 3: Building the Team

1. Bain, K. (2011). *What the Best College Teachers Do*. Cambridge, MA: Harvard University Press.
2. Ludmerer, K. M. (1999). *Time to Heal: American Medical Education from the Turn of the Century to the Era of Managed Care*. New York: Oxford University Press.
3. Ramani, S. (2003). Twelve tips to improve bedside teaching. *Medical Teacher*, *25*(2), 112–115.
4. Kendra, T. (2011). Bo Schembechler's legendary "The Team" speech still rings true today in high school football. *The Muskegon Chronicle*. Retrieved from August 24, 2011, http://www.mlive.com/sports/muskegon/index.ssf/2011/08/bo_schembechlers_legendary_the.html.
5. Mann, K. V. (2011). Theoretical perspectives in medical education: Past experience and future possibilities. *Medical Education*, *45*(1), 60–68.

6. Weinstein, D. (2011). Ensuring an effective physician workforce for the United States: Recommendations for graduate medical education to meet the needs of the public. Content and format of GME (2nd of two conferences), Atlanta, GA. May, 2011. Josiah Macy Jr. Foundation.
7. Sutcliffe, K. M., Lewton, E., & Rosenthal, M. M. (2004). Communication failures: An insidious contributor to medical mishaps. *Academic Medicine, 79*(2), 186–194.

Chapter 4: A Safe, Supportive Environment

1. Mann, K. V. (2011). Theoretical perspectives in medical education: Past experience and future possibilities. *Medical Education, 45*(1), 60–68.
2. Sutkin, G., Wagner, E., Harris, I., & Schiffer, R. (2008). What makes a good clinical teacher in medicine? A review of the literature. *Academic Medicine, 83*(5), 452–466.

Chapter 5: Bedside and Beyond

1. Shankel, S. W., & Mazzaferri, E. L. (1986). Teaching the resident in internal medicine: Present practices and suggestions for the future. *Journal of the American Medical Association, 256*(6), 725–729.
2. Block, L., Habicht, R., Wu, A. W., Desai, S. V., Wang, K., Silva, K. N., . . . Feldman, L. (2013). In the wake of the 2003 and 2011 duty hours regulations, how do internal medicine interns spend their time? *Journal of General Internal Medicine, 28*(8), 1042–1047.
3. Ahmed, K., & El-Bagir, M. (2002). What is happening to bedside clinical teaching? *Medical Education, 36*(12), 1185–1188.
4. Easy auscultation. MedEdu LLC. (2015). Retrieved from http://www.easyauscultation.com/egophony.
5. Gladstone, D. J., Spring, M., Dorian, P., Panzov, V., Thorpe, K. E., Hall, J., . . . Côté, R. (2014). Atrial fibrillation in patients with cryptogenic stroke. *New England Journal of Medicine, 370*(26), 2467–2477.
6. Saint, S. (2010). *Saint-Frances Guide: Clinical Clerkship in Inpatient Medicine.* (3rd edition). Baltimore, MD: Lippincott Williams & Wilkins.

Chapter 6: How to Think About Thinking

1. Eva, K. W. (2005). What every teacher needs to know about clinical reasoning. *Medical Education, 39*(1), 98–106.
2. Irby, D. M. (2014). Excellence in clinical teaching: Knowledge transformation and development required. *Medical Education, 48*(8), 776–784.
3. Centor, R. M., & Willett, L. L. (2008). Becoming a better ward attending: Ten modifiable behaviors. ACP Hospitalist. Retrieved from http://www.acphospitalist.org/archives/2008/05/attending.htm.
4. Introduction to the Socratic method and its effect on critical thinking. 2009–2015. Retrieved from http://www.socratic-method.net/.
5. Bain, K. (2011). *What the Best College Teachers Do.* Cambridge, MA: Harvard University Press.

Chapter 7: Role Models

1. Wright, S., Wong, A., & Newill, C. (1997). The impact of role models on medical students. *Journal of General Internal Medicine, 12*(1), 53–56.
2. Branch, Jr. W. T., Kern, D., Haidet, P., Weissmann, P., Gracey, C. F., Mitchell, G., & Inui, T. (2001). Teaching the human dimensions of care in clinical settings. *Journal of the American Medical Association, 286*(9), 1067–1074.
3. Detsky, A. S., & Verma, A. A. (2012). A new model for medical education: Celebrating restraint. *Journal of the American Medical Association, 308*(13), 1329–1330.

Chapter 8: The Sacred Act of Healing

1. Institute of Medicine, Committee on Quality of Health Care in America. (2001). *Crossing the Quality Chasm: A New Health System for the 21st Century.* Report No.: 0309073227. Washington, D.C.: National Academy Press.
2. Peabody, F. W. (1927). The care of the patient. *Journal of the American Medical Association, 88*(12), 877–882.

INDEX

physical examination, 98–99
preparation, charts and labs,
58, 59f, 60–63, 100–101, 116
role modeling, 28, 83–93, 98
(*See also* Role models)
Heuristics, teaching, 80
Hidden curriculum, 86–88
Hirschtick, Robert, MD, 122, 122f
Hospitalists, 12
Hospital personnel
relations, 27–29
Hospitals. *See* Teaching hospitals
House officers, 20–21
Humor, 7, 15–16
gallows, 48, 92
with learners, 15–16, 46–48, 47f
with patients and families, 92,
96–97, 102–103, 105
self-deprecating, 16
Hunt, Daniel P., MD, 123, 123f
Hypotheticals, 77–78

Identification, with learner, 39
Improvement, self-, 15, 86–87
Inclusion, team member, 22–23
Independent thinking,
fostering, 40
Index cards, 70
Individualized patient care, 55
Internship hours, 51–52
Interruptions, 35
Intuitive care, 74–75
Irby, David M., 30, 72, 118, 134

Journal articles, 68

Kneeling, bedside, 106, 105f
Knowledge
acquisition, 24
of patients, 58, 59f, 60–63,
100–101, 116
sharing, 14, 14f

Learner. *See also specific topics*
assistance, proactive, 38
physician as, 114
Learning
from current to next
patient, 54, 63
eagerness for, 39
hours, reduced, 4
knowledge acquisition, 24
team-based, 24–25, 114
Learning–stress curve, 76, 76f
Lightheartedness, 7, 15–16
Listening to patient, 105–106
Love of sharing knowledge, 14, 14f
Love of teaching, 13
Ludmerer, Kenneth, 21, 31, 118, 132

Maycock, Robert, MD, 124, 124f
Mba, Benjamin, MBBS, MRCP,
125, 125f
McGee, Steven, MD, 126, 126f
Medical errors, 4, 45–46
Medical schools
annual graduates, 2
history, 20–21
Mistakes
attendees, 90
attendings, 40–41, 43
as learning opportunities, 33
Mnemonic, 69

Non-question question, 78–79
Nurses, respecting, 28

Openness, 35, 36f
Outpatient care, 107
Ownership, 99

Papadakis, Maxine, 10
Patient-centered care and
teaching, 3, 95–96, 101,
104–107, 105f, 115–116